Medical Device Quality Assurance and Regulatory Compliance

Medical Device Quality Assurance and Regulatory Compliance

Richard C. Fries

Datex-Ohmeda
Madison, Wisconsin

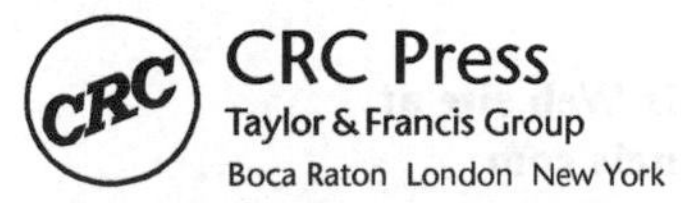

CRC Press is an imprint of the
Taylor & Francis Group, an **informa** business

CRC Press
Taylor & Francis Group
6000 Broken Sound Parkway NW, Suite 300
Boca Raton, FL 33487-2742

First issued in paperback 2019

ISBN-13: 978-0-367-40036-1

Visit the Taylor & Francis Web site at
http://www.taylorandfrancis.com

and the CRC Press Web site at
http://www.crcpress.com

To

Helen Grenier

whose lifelong committment to education

has been a constant inspiration

Preface

Medical device manufacturers establish and follow quality systems to ensure their products are safe, effective, and reliable for their intended use and consistently meet applicable specifications and requirements. To assist the manufacturer in this goal, standards for quality systems have been established worldwide. In addition, individual countries or groups of countries have developed regulations that must be met prior to importing a product to that country.

In the United States, the quality systems for products regulated by the Food and Drug Administration (FDA) are known as the Quality System regulation. In addition, the Safe Medical Devices Act of 1990 provided FDA with the authority to add preproduction design controls to the regulations. The FDA has also enacted regulations regarding submission of data prior to making a device available in the marketplace.

Internationally, the ISO 9000 series addresses quality systems for all manufacturers. Working group 1 of ISO Technical Committee 210 has developed standards (ISO 13485 and ISO 13488), which apply ISO 9001 to medical devices. EN 46000 is a European standard that specifically addresses medical devices. Recently, the ISO 14000 series of standards were published to address environmental issues for all manufacturers.

In 1992, the Global Harmonization Task Force (GHTF) was formed in an effort to harmonize regulatory requirements for the medical device industry. The GHTF consists of representatives for the Canadian Ministry of Health and Welfare, the Japanese Ministry of Health and Welfare, the FDA, industry members from the European Union, Australia, Canada, Japan, the United States, and a few delegates from observing countries.

The world of quality assurance and regulatory compliance can be one of confusion and bewilderment. This book attempts to give some direction to the medical device manufacturer so that compliance activity becomes a standard part of the product development process. The primary goal of this text is to acquaint the developer of medical devices with the basic concepts and major issues of medical quality assurance and regulatory documents, to describe the requirements listed in these documents, and to provide strategies for compliance to these requirements. To achieve this goal, this book is divided into 5 sections.

Section 1 is an overview of the various quality assurance and regulatory requirements. It discusses the history of the FDA, the European Economic Community, and the Global Harmonization Task Force.

Section 2 discusses in detail the quality system standards. The ISO 9000 series of standards is reviewed, followed by an in-depth discussion of each requirement, and a strategy for meeting those requirements. Discussions include choosing a standard from the series, getting the company ready for the auditor, choosing a notified body, and surviving the audit. Section 2 concludes with a discussion of the ISO 14000 series of standards in the same depth.

While Section 2 looked at the process, Section 3 investigates the product. Standards are discussed that deal specifically with medical devices, including EN 46000, ISO 13485, and ISO 13488. EN 46000 is a standard that addresses the product development process. After an overview of the standard, this section looks at the individual requirements of the standard and then discusses a strategy for meeting those requirements. ISO 13485 and 13488 are recent standards developed to address ISO 9001 requirements for medical devices. Many in Europe suggest that eventually, these documents will replace EN 46000. The requirements of ISO 13485 and 13488 are examined in detail, followed by a strategy for compliance.

Section 4 deals with Regulatory compliance. Each of the Medical Device Directives is discussed, followed by a detailed discussion of requirements and a strategy for compliance. This is followed by a similar discussion of the new Quality System Regulation requirements and the requirements for product submittals prior to product introduction. These discussions will include current issues the FDA is attempting to deal with, including third party approvals.

Section 5 consists of various appendices listing standards organizations, Quality System registrars/Notified Bodies, regulatory agencies, various FDA offices, consultants and training organizations, and testing organizations. The final appendix is a glossary of terms.

Knowledge of the quality assurance and regulatory requirements is an essential part of every medical device development process. Being able to comply with the requirements is essential to the financial success of the manufacturer. It is hoped this text will be an invaluable resource in establishing standards and regulatory compliance as a vital part of every medical device manufacturer's operation.

I am deeply indebted to many people for their encouragement, help, and constructive criticism in the preparation of this book. I want to thank Tina Juneau and Chuck Morreale who reviewed the chapters and provided fresh insight. I want to thank Eric Stannard at Marcel Dekker, Inc., whose expertise and humor made the job of editing this book tolerable. Mostly, I want to thank my wife, June, who constantly encouraged me and who sacrificed much quality time during the preparation and editing that we otherwise would have spent together.

Richard C. Fries

Contents

Section 1

Standards and Regulations Background

Chapter 1

Quality Assurance and Regulatory Compliance

As a result of revolutionary changes that have occurred around the world, we are part of an inevitable phenomenon: globalization of the economy. Internationalization of competition, deregulation of world trade, the boom of the information economy, and the management revolution move more and more companies to change the way they do business, the way they think, and the way they manage. They are adapting to the new reality to ensure their present survival and future prosperity. Many are reconfiguring their organizations and adopting new political, technical, and cultural values. Business leaders are revolutionizing their management thinking and implementing strategic information management, total quality management, empowerment, reengineering, policy deployment, cross-functional management, activity-based management, and environmental management. Quality may be the biggest competitive issue of the new century.

1.1 Quality Assurance

At the start of this century, mass production and the evolution of technology quickly rendered unit inspection costly, ineffective, or inapplicable. This period was marked by the birth of statistical sampling for inspection and acceptance of the product at receiving and shipping. This inspection method, based on attributes that permit classification of lots as good or bad, did not preclude the delivery of a certain percentage of defective products to the buyer. In 1924, at Bell Laboratories in the United States, Walter Shewhart invented the control chart as a tool for measuring process variations. In general, these statistical control methods were limited to process control and to product inspection, and served to detect non-quality.

In the 1950s, the United States introduced a new procurement concept in the military sector. Instead of gathering enough qualified inspectors to examine large quantities of goods or parts that were physically impossible to inspect, Department of Defense (DOD) experts advocated quality assurance by establishing the MIL-Q-9858 standard. For the first time in history, this quality program detailed contractual specifications for procurement. In the early 1960s, this contractual philosophy appeared in the United Kingdom in the Polaris program.

During this period, quality assurance was focused on the supplier. The idea consisted not only of inspecting parts, but of assuring that the supplier was perfectly organized. To implement this idea, purchasers required a set of preventive measures and evidence of their application from suppliers before ordering. However, the quality assurance field lacked clear distinctions and definitions of concepts such as inspection, quality control, statistical control, internal and external quality assurance, quality management, and total quality management.

Today, businesses are changing from the mass production model to the mass customization model and quality assurance is focused on the customer. This renewed concept consists of establishing guidelines, measures, and rules within a quality system that encompasses the majority of a company's activities. The key is to prevent, detect, and resolve problems of non-quality with trained employees and to demonstrate the effectiveness of the chosen measure in order to attract customer satisfaction. Quality Assurance includes inspection and statistical quality controls as a means of detection and sometimes even as a prevention tool. Quality management, as fine-tuned by quality leaders such as W. Edward Deming, Joseph Juran, and Kaoru Ishikawa, consists in the company elaborating its own quality policy and vision for customer satisfaction. Quality management requires-top leadership commitment and a customer-focused approach that goes far beyond a service of quality assurance. In constant evolution, this concept has developed into Total Quality Management (TQM). It integrates the employees', the customers', and the owners' satisfaction while also respecting the environment and society.

1.2 Regulation

Medical devices are an extraordinarily heterogeneous category of products. The term *medical device* includes such technologically simple articles as ice bags and tongue depressors. On the other end of the spectrum, very sophisticated articles such as pacemakers and surgical lasers are also medical devices. Perhaps it is this diversity of products coupled with the sheer number of different devices that makes the development of an effective and efficient regulatory scheme a unique challenge for the Congress and the Food and Drug Administration (FDA) in the United States and the European Commission (EC) in Europe.

1.2.1 Regulation in the United States

Historically, medical devices have been neglected from a legislative and regulatory perspective. In the early 1900s, Congressional attention focused on food and drugs. The Pure Food and Drug Act of 1906 was passed to prohibit the distribution of adulterated or misbranded food and drugs to interstate commerce. This legislation, however, did not include any provisions to enable the Food and Drug Administration to regulate medical devices. Thus, legitimate and fraudulent medical devices were freely marketed without any effective check on the safety of these articles or the accuracy of their claims.

The most significant rationale for authorizing the FDA to regulate medical devices was the mounting level of consumer fraud. In the years preceding the Federal Food, Drug, and Cosmetic Act of 1938, medical devices were marketed that touted false therapeutic claims. Many of these devices were patently harmful. Others, by virtue of their bogus therapeutic claims, delayed consumers from seeking proper medical attention. Thus, a growing concern evolved - the public welfare was in jeopardy unless a mechanism was established to regulate the safety and reliability of medical devices.

It was not until 1938, when the Pure Food and Drug Act of 1906 underwent extensive revision, that the Congress expressly empowered the federal government to regulate medical devices. The Federal Food, Drug and Cosmetic Act of 1938 expanded the FDA's regulatory control over food and drugs and extended the agency's authority to include medical devices and cosmetics.

The FDA's regulatory authority over medical devices remained unchanged until the mid-1970s. In the late 1960s and early 1970s, there was some interest expressed by administrative officials and members of Congress in improving the regulatory framework for medical devices. Although some of this interest culminated in device regulation bills, formal legislation was not enacted until May, 1976. The Medical Device Amendments to the Federal Food, Drug, and Cosmetic Act, of 1976, established an intricate statutory framework to enable the FDA to regulate nearly every aspect of medical devices, from testing through marketing.

1.2.2 Regulation in Europe

The European Community's program on the completion of the Internal Market has, as the primary objective for medical devices, to ensure Community-wide free circulation of products. The only means to establish such free circulation, in view of quite divergent national systems, regulations governing medical devices, and existing trade barriers, was to adopt legislation for the Community, by which the health and safety of patients, users, and third persons would be ensured through a harmonized set of device related protection requirements. Devices meeting the requirements and sold to members of the Community are identified by means of a CE mark.

Because of the diversity of current national medical device standards, attempts to introduce mutual recognition of device approvals to reconcile the different regimes proved to be fruitless. The European Commission eventually decided that totally new EC legislation, covering all medical devices was needed.

The Active Implantable Medical Devices Directive adopted by the Community legislator in 1990 and the Medical Devices Directive in 1993 cover more than 80% of medical devices for use with human beings. The In-Vitro Diagnostic Medical Devices Directive, which came into force in 1997, addresses the remaining devices. After a period of transition, i.e., a period during which the laws implementing a Directive co-exist with pre-existing national laws, these directives exhaustively govern the conditions for placing medical devices on the market. Through the agreements on the European Economic Area (EEA), the relevant requirements and procedures are the same for all European Community member states and European Free Trade Association (EFTA) countries that belong to the EEA, an economic area comprising more than 380 million people.

1.3 Standards

The degree to which formal standards and procedures are applied to product development varies from company to company. In many cases, standards are dictated by customers or regulatory mandate. In other situations, standards are self-imposed. If formal standards do exist, an assurance activity must be established to guarantee that they are being followed. An assessment of compliance to standards may be conducted as part of a formal technical review or by audit.

Standards simplify communication, promote consistency and uniformity, and eliminate the need to invent yet another solution to the same problem. They are a way of preserving proven practices above and beyond the inevitable staff changes within organizations. Standards, whether official or merely agreed upon, are especially important when talking to customers and suppliers, but it is easy to underestimate their importance when dealing with different departments and disciplines within our own organization.

1.3.1 Standards in the United States

Standards are important in that they impact our industry in many ways. Most of the standards activity relevant to the medical device, diagnostic product, and health care information systems industry, falls into one or more of the four following types:

- regulatory
- national voluntary consensus
- foreign national
- international.

Regulatory standards are those that generally have some basis in law. National voluntary standards are the work products of groups. Foreign national standards are like our own national regulatory and voluntary standards except that they are for other countries. International standards are the attempts by countries to try to reduce the differences in national standards through organizations such as the International Organization for Standardization (ISO) and the International Electrotechnical Commission (IEC).

People who work on medical device standards have been conditioned to think only in terms of voluntary and regulatory standards. While that may be a useful distinction in law, in practice, the distinctions blur because most standards fit into a gray area. From a practical point of view it does not matter very much if a standard is labeled mandatory or voluntary. There are examples of regulatory agency standards being promoted as guidelines and voluntary standards being used as mandatory requirements.

The American National Standards Institute's (ANSI) 1987 *Summary Annual Report of Medical Device Standards Board Activities* identifies over 700 voluntary medical device standards completed or under development. These standards cover everything from needles, syringes, and thermometers to diagnostic test kits, electrical safety, and laboratory computers. Some of these standards are clearly defined and cover only a specific device. Others, however, are so broad - on sterilization, for example - that they cover whole classes of medical devices.

1.3.1.1 Software Standards

There are a myriad of software standards to assist the developer in designing and documenting his program. The Institute of Electrical and Electronic Engineers' (IEEE) standards cover documentation through all phases of design. Military standards describe how software is to be designed and developed for military use. There are also standards on software quality and reliability to assist developers in preparing a quality program. The international community has produced standards, primarily dealing with software safety. In each case, the standard is a voluntary document that has been developed to provide guidelines for designing, developing, testing, and documenting a software program.

In the United States, the FDA is responsible for assuring the device utilizing software or the software as a device is safe and effective for its intended use. The FDA has produced several drafts of reviewer guidelines, auditor guidelines, software policy, and Quality System regulations addressing both device and process software. In addition, guidelines for FDA reviewers have been prepared as well as training programs for inspectors and reviewers. The Quality System Regulation addresses software as part of the design phase.

The United States is ahead of other countries in establishing guidelines for medical software development. There is, however, movement within several international organizations to develop regulations and guidelines for software and software controlled devices. For example, ISO 9000-3, *Quality management and quality assurance standards - Part 3: Guidelines for the application of ISO 9001 to the development, supply and maintenance of software,* specifically addresses software development in addition to what is contained in ISO 9001. The Canadian Standards Association (CSA) addresses software issues in four standards covering new and previously developed software in critical and non-critical applications. IEC has a software document currently in development.

1.3.2 International Standards

Internationally, standards may be defined as:

> A technical specification or other document available to the public, drawn up with the cooperation and consensus or general approval of all interests affected by it, based on the consolidated results of science, technology and experience, aimed at the promotion of optimum community benefits and approved by a body on the national, regional, or international level.

While this definition goes some way to saying what a standard is, it says nothing about the subject matter or purpose, apart from stating that the objectives of the standard must in some way be tied to community benefits.
Standards, however, have a definite subject matter. They include:

- to standardize particular processes,
- to provide a consistent and complete definition of a commodity or process,
- to record good practice regarding the development process associated with the production of commodities,
- to encode good practice for the specification, design, manufacture, testing, maintenance, and operation of commodities.

One of the primary requirements of a standard is that it be produced in such a way that conformance to the standard can be unambiguously determined. A standard is devalued if conformance can not be easily determined or if the standard is so loosely worded that it becomes a matter of debate and conjecture as to whether the requirements of the standard have been met.

Standards also exist in various types:

- De facto and de jure standards. These are usually associated with the prevailing commercial interests in the market place. These de facto standards are often eventually subject to the standardization process.

- Reference models. These provide a framework within which standards can be formulated.
- Product versus process standards. Some standards relate to specific products while others relate to the process used to produce products.
- Codes of practice, guidelines, and specifications. These terms relate to the manner in which a standard may be enforced. Codes of practice and guidelines reflect ways of working that are deemed to be *good* or *desirable*, but for which conformance is difficult to determine. Specifications are far more precise and conformance can be determined by analysis or test.
- Prospective and retrospective standards. It is clearly undesirable to develop a standard before the subject matter is well understood scientifically, technically, and through practice. However, it may be desirable to develop a standard alongside the evolving technology.

1.4 Coping with Increased Quality Assurance and Regulatory Issues

A manufacturer has several options available for coping with a changing QA and regulatory environment. These range from participating in shaping the new standards and regulations, to responding to them upon completion. Ignoring them is not considered a viable option.

It is important for manufacturers to be involved in the development process for a new standard or regulation. By being part of the process, they can minimize the impact of the new requirements on their development of a product. They can also present knowledgeable inputs to the discussion, based on experience, that will make the standard or regulation more effective.

Standards and regulatory agencies are very keen to inputs from those subject to the standard or regulation. Agencies are interested in developing good working relationships with organizations that are affected by their rules and regulations. It is in the interest of both parties to develop standards and regulations that are meaningful, effective, and do not present an extraordinary burden.

References

Appler, William D. and Gaile L. McMann, "Medical Device Regulation: The Big Picture," in *The Medical Device Industry: Science, Technology, and Regulation in a Competitive Environment.* New York: Marcel Dekker, Inc., 1990.

American National Standards Institute, *Summary Annual Report of Medical Device Standards Board Activities.* New York: American National Standards Institute, 1987,

Deming, W. Edward, *Out of the Crisis.* Cambridge, MA: MIT Center for Advanced Engineering Studies, 1986.

Department of Defense, *MIL-Q-9858.* April 4, 1959.

Fries, Richard C., *Reliable Design of Medical Devices.* New York: Marcel Dekker, Inc., 1997.

Higson, Gordon R., *The Medical Devices Directives - A Manufacturers' Handbook.* Brussels: Medical Technology Consultants Europe Ltd., 1993.

Naisbitt, John, *Global Paradox.* New York: Avon Books, 1995.

Olsson, John E., "Trends in International Regulations and Their Growing Impact." In *The Medical Device Industry.* Norman F. Estrin, editor. New York: Marcel Dekker, Inc., 1990.

Shepard, Stephen, "Defining the Q-word," in *Business Week*, Special Issue, 1991.

Todorov, Branimir, *ISO 9000 Required: Your Worldwide Passport to Customer Confidence.* Portland, OR: Productivity Press, 1996.

Willingmyre, George T., "Industry's Role in Standards Development," in *The Medical Device Industry - Science, Technology, and Regulation in a Competitive Environment.* New York: Marcel Dekker, Inc., 1990.

Chapter 2

The FDA

Regulation of medical devices is intended to protect consumer's health and safety by attempting to ensure that marketed products are effective and safe. Prior to 1976, the FDA had limited authority over medical devices under the Food, Drug, and Cosmetic Act of 1938. Beginning in 1968, Congress established a radiation control program to authorize the establishment of standards for electronic products, including medical and dental radiology equipment. From the early 1960s to 1975, concern over devices increased and six United States Presidential messages were given to encourage medical device legislation.

In 1969, the Department of Health, Education, and Welfare appointed a special committee (the Cooper Committee) to review the scientific literature associated with medical devices. The Committee estimated that over a 10 year period, 10,000 injuries were associated with medical devices, of which 731 resulted in death. The majority of problems were associated with three device types: artificial heart valves, cardiac pacemakers, and intrauterine contraceptive devices. There activities culminated in passage of the Medical Devices Amendments of 1976.

Devices marketed after 1976 are subject to full regulation unless they are found substantially equivalent to a device already on the market in 1976. By the end of 1981, only about 300 of the 17,000 products submitted for clearance to the FDA after 1976 had been found not substantially equivalent.

2.1 History of the FDA

In 1906, the Food and Drug Administration enacted its first regulations addressing public health. While these regulations did not address medical devices per se, they did establish a foundation for future regulations. It was not until 1938, with the passage of the Federal Food, Drug and Cosmetic Act (FFD&C) that the FDA was authorized, for the first time, to regulate medical devices. This act provided for regulation of adulterated or misbranded drugs, cosmetics, and devices that were entered into interstate commerce. A medical device could be marketed without being federally reviewed and approved.

In the years following World War II, the FDA focused much of the attention on drugs and cosmetics. Over-the-counter drugs became regulated in 1961. In 1962, the FDA began requesting safety and efficacy data on new drugs and cosmetics.

By the mid-1960s, it became clear that the provisions of the FFD&C Act were not adequate to regulate the complex medical devices of the times to ensure both patient and user safety. Thus, in 1969, the Cooper Committee was formed to examine the problems associated with medical devices and to develop concepts for new regulations.

In 1976, with input from the Cooper Committee, the FDA created the Medical Device Amendments to the FFD&C Act, which were subsequently signed into law. The purpose of the amendments was to ensure that medical devices were safe, effective, and properly labeled for their intended use. To accomplish this mandate, the amendments provided the FDA with the authority to regulate devices during most phases of their development, testing, production, distribution, and use. This marked the first time the FDA clearly distinguished between devices and drugs. Regulatory requirements were derived from this 1976 law.

In 1978, with the authority granted the FDA by the amendments, the Good Manufacturing Practices (GMP) were promulgated. The GMP represents a quality assurance program intended to control the manufacturing, packaging, storage, distribution, and installation of medical devices. This regulation was intended to allow only safe and effective devices to reach the market place. It is this regulation that has the greatest effect on the medical device industry. It allows the FDA to inspect a company's operations and take action on any noted deficiencies, including prohibition of device shipment.

Recent regulations specific to medical devices are the Medical Device Reporting (MDR) regulation of 1984, the Device Reconditioner/Rebuilder (DRR) regulation of 1988, the Safe Medical Devices Act of 1992, and the Quality System Regulation of 1997.

2.2 Registration and Listing

Under Section 510 of the FFD&C Act, every person engaged in the manufacture, preparation, propagation, compounding, or processing of a device shall register their name, place of business and such establishment. This includes manufacturers of devices and components, repackers, relabelers, as well as initial distributors of imported devices. Those not required to register include manufacturers of raw materials, licensed practitioners, manufacturers of devices for use solely in research or teaching, warehousers, manufacturers of veterinary devices, and those who only dispense devices, such as pharmacies.

Upon registration, the FDA issues a device registration number. A change in the ownership or corporate structure of the firm, the location, or person designated as the official correspondent must be communicated to the FDA device registration and listing branch within 30 days. Registration must be done when first beginning to manufacture medical devices and must be updated yearly.

Section 510 of the FFD&C Act also requires all manufacturers to list the medical devices they market. Listing includes not only informing the FDA of products manufactured, but also providing the agency with copies of labeling and advertising. Listing must be done when first beginning to manufacture a product. Device listing need to be updated when one or more of the following occurs:

- a device is introduced into commercial distribution with a classification name not currently listed with the FDA
- the intended use of a listed device changes in such a way that would result in its being more appropriately classified under a different classification name
- the marketing of all devices having the same classification name is discontinued by the company

- a commercial distribution of devices identified by a previously discontinued classification name is resumed by the company
- a change occurs in the owner or operator, registration number, establishment name, or establishment type.

Foreign firms that market products in the United States are permitted but not required to register, and are required to list. Foreign devices that are not listed are not permitted to enter the country.

Registration and listing provides the FDA with information about the identity of manufacturers and the products they make. This information enables the agency to schedule inspections of facilities and also to follow up on problems. When the FDA learns about a safety defect in a particular type of device, it can use the listing information to notify all manufacturers of those devices about that defect.

2.3 Device Classification

A medical device is any article or health care product intended for use in the diagnosis of disease or other condition or for use in the care, treatment, or prevention of disease that does not achieve any of its primary intended purposes by chemical action or by being metabolized.

From 1962, when Congress passed the last major drug law revision, and first attempted to include devices, until 1976 when device laws were finally written, there were almost constant congressional hearings. Testimony was presented by medical and surgical specialty groups, industry, basic biomedical sciences, and various government agencies, including the FDA. All of the viewpoints and arguments that we hear today were proposed, and considered in public discussion. Nearly two dozen bills were rejected as either inadequate or inappropriate.

The Cooper Committee concluded that the many inherent and important differences between drugs and devices necessitated a regulatory plan specifically adapted to devices. They recognized that some degree of risk is inherent in the development of many devices. They also realized that:

- all hazards cannot be eliminated
- there is often little or no prior experience on which to base judgments about safety and effectiveness

- that devices undergo performance improvement modifications during the course of clinical trials
- that results also depend upon the skill of the user.

They therefore rejected the drug-based approach and created a new system for evaluating devices. All devices were placed into classes based upon the degree of risk posed by each individual device and its intended use. The Pre-Market Notification Process (510(k)) and the Pre-Market Approval Application (PMAA) became the regulatory pathways for device approval. The Investigational Device Exemption (IDE) became the mechanism to establish safety and efficacy in clinical studies for PMAAs.

2.3.1 Class I Devices

Class I devices were defined in 1976 as non-life sustaining devices, whose failure posed no risk to life, and thus required no need for performance standards. Basic standards, however, such as premarket notification (510(k)), registration, device listing, good manufacturing practices (GMP), and proper record keeping are all required. Nonetheless, the FDA has exempted many of the simpler Class I devices from some or all of these requirements. For example, tongue depressors and stethoscopes are both Class I devices; both are exempt from GMP, tongue depressors are exempt from 510(k) filing, whereas stethoscopes are not.

2.3.2 Class II Devices

Class II devices were also defined as non-life sustaining devices. However, they must not only comply with the basic standards for Class I devices, but must meet specific controls or performance standards. For example, sphygmomanometers, although not essential for life, must meet standards of accuracy and reproducibility. Class II devices must also have premarket notification information submitted prior to marketing.

Premarket notification is documentation submitted by a manufacturer that notifies the FDA that a device is about to be marketed. It assists the agency in making a determination about whether the device is "substantially equivalent" to a previously marketed predecessor device. As provided for in section 510(k) of the Food, Drug, and Cosmetic Act, the FDA can clear a device for marketing on the basis of premarket notification that the device is substantially equivalent to a pre-1976 predecessor device. The decision is based on premarket notification information that is provided by the manufacturer including the intended use, physical composition, specifications of the device, and risk analysis. Additional data usually submitted includes environmental testing, verification and validation results, and compatibility studies.

The premarket notification or 510(k) process was designed to give manufacturers the opportunity to obtain rapid market approval of these noncritical devices by providing evidence that their device is "substantially equivalent" to a device that is already marketed. The device must have the same intended use and the same or equally safe and effective technological characteristics as a predicate device.

The Safe Medical Device Act of 1990 and the Amendments of 1992 attempted to take advantage of what had been learned since 1976. The regulations gave both the FDA and manufacturers greater leeway by permitting down-classification of many devices, including some life supporting and life sustaining devices previously in Class III. This was based on the fact that reasonable assurance of safety and effectiveness could be obtained by application of "Special Controls" such as performance standards, post market surveillance, guidelines, and patient and device registries.

2.3.3 Class III Devices

Class III devices were defined in 1976 as either sustaining or supporting life so that their failure is life threatening. For example, heart valves, pacemakers and PCTA balloon catheters are all Class III devices. Class III devices almost always require a PMAA, a long and complicated task fraught with many pitfalls, that has caused the greatest confusion and dissatisfaction for both industry and the FDA.

The new regulations permit the FDA to use data contained in four prior PMAs for a specific device, that demonstrate safety and effectiveness, to approve future PMA applications by establishing performance standards or actual reclassification. Composition and manufacturing methods which companies wish to keep as proprietary secrets are excluded. Advisory Medical panel review is now elective.

However, for PMAAs that continue to be required, all of the basic requirements for Class I and II devices must be provided, plus failure mode analysis, animal tests, toxicology studies, and then finally human clinical studies, directed to establish safety and efficacy under an IDE.

It is necessary that preparation of the PMA must actually begin years before it will be submitted. It is only after the company has the results of all of the laboratory testing, pre-clinical animal testing, failure mode analysis and manufacturing standards on their final design, that their proof of safety and efficacy can begin, in the form of a clinical study under an IDE.

At this point the manufacturer must not only have settled on a specific, fixed design for his device, but with his marketing and clinical consultants must also have decided on what the indications, contraindications, and warnings for use will be. The clinical study must be carefully designed to support these claims.

Section 520(g) of the Federal Food, Drug, and Cosmetic Act, as amended, authorizes the FDA to grant an IDE to a researcher using a device in studies undertaken to develop safety and effectiveness data for that device when such studies involve human subjects. An approved IDE application permits a device that would otherwise be subject to marketing clearance to be shipped lawfully for the purpose of conducting a clinical study. An approved IDE also exempts a device from certain sections of the Act. All new significant risk devices not granted substantial equivalence under the 510(k) section of the Act must pursue clinical testing under an IDE.

An Institutional Review Board (IRB) is any board, committee, or other group formally designated by an institution to review, approve the initiation of, and conduct periodic review of biomedical research involving human subjects. The primary purpose of the review is to ensure the protection of the rights and welfare of human subjects. Any human research covered by federal regulation will not be funded unless it has been reviewed by an IRB. The fundamental purpose of an IRB is to ensure that research activities are conducted in an ethica and legal manner. Specifically, IRBs are expected to ensure that each of the basic elements of informed consent, as defined by regulation, are included in the document presented to the research participant for signature or verbal approval.

2.4 Medical Device Submissions

Medical device submissions may be of separate types:

- 510(k)
- Premarket Approval (PMA)
- Investigational Device Exemption (IDE).

Under section 510(k) of the Federal Food, Drug, and Cosmetic Act, a person who intends to introduce a device into commercial distribution is required to submit a premarket notification, or 510(k), to the FDA at least 90 days before commercial distribution is to begin. The FDA may then issue an order of substantial equivalence, only upon making a determination that the device to be introduced into commercial distribution is as safe and effective as a legally marketed device.

Premarket Approval (PMA) is an approval application for a Class III medical device, including all information submitted with or incorporated by reference. The purpose of the regulation is to establish an efficient and thorough device review process to facilitate the approval of PMAs for devices that have been shown to be safe and effective for their intended use and that otherwise meet the statutory criteria for approval, while ensuring the disapproval of PMAs for devices that have not been shown to be safe and effective or that do not otherwise meet the statutory criteria for approval.

The purpose of the Investigational Device Exemption (IDE) regulation is to encourage the discovery and development of useful devices intended for human use while protecting the public health. It provides the procedures for the conduct of clinical investigations of devices. An approved IDE permits a device to be shipped lawfully for the purpose of conducting investigations of the device without complying with a performance standard or having marketing clearance.

2.5 Medical Device Reporting

On July 31, 1996, the new Medical Device Reporting (MDR) regulation became effective for user facilities and device manufacturers. The MDR regulation provides a mechanism for the Food and Drug Administration and manufacturers to identify and monitor significant adverse events involving medical devices. The goals are to detect and correct problems in a timely manner. Although the requirements of the regulation can be enforced through legal sanctions authorized by the Federal Food, Drug and Cosmetic Act, FDA relies on the goodwill and cooperation of all affected groups to accomplish the objectives of the regulation.

The statutory authority for the MDR regulation is section 519 of the FD&C Act as amended by the Safe Medical Devices Act (SMDA) of 1990. The SMDA requires user facilities to report:

- device-related deaths to the FDA and the device manufacturer,

- device-related serious injuries and serious illnesses to the manufacturer, or to FDA if the manufacturer is not known,
- submit to FDA on a semiannual basis a summary of all reports submitted during that period.

2.6 Quality System Regulation

Current good manufacturing practice requirements are set forth in the Quality System Regulation of 1996. The requirements govern the methods used in, and the facilities and controls used for, the design, manufacture, packaging, labeling, storage, installation, and servicing of all finished devices intended for human use. The requirements are intended to ensure that finished devices will be safe and effective and otherwise in compliance with the Federal Food, Drug, and Cosmetic Act by establishing basic requirements applicable to manufacturers of finished medical devices. The regulation establishes for the first time design control requirements. The format of the regulation is very similar to that of ISO 9001.

The regulation is applicable to any finished device intended for human use that is manufactured, imported, or offered for import in any state or territory of the United States, the District of Columbia, or the Commonwealth of Puerto Rico.

The regulation went into effect June 1, 1997. A grace period has been granted until June 14, 1998, the same day the grace period for the Medical Device Directives ends. During the grace period, the FDA may inspect a manufacturer's facilities to the Quality System Regulation, but may not list any findings on the form 483 or bring sanctions against a manufacturer for non-compliances to the Quality System Regulation.

2.7 The FDA Inspection

The FDA's power to inspect originates in Section 704 of the Federal Food, Drug, and Cosmetic Act. This provision allows FDA officials to inspect any factory, warehouse, or establishment in which devices are manufactured, processed, packed or held, for introduction into interstate commerce of after such introduction. In addition to the "establishments" specification, FDA is permitted to enter any vehicle used to transport or hold regulated products for export or in interstate commerce. The inspection power is specifically extended to medical device manufacturers by Sections 519 and 520 of the Federal Food, Drug, and Cosmetic Act.

Every FDA inspector is authorized by law to inspect all equipment that is used in the manufacturing process. Furthermore, investigators may examine finished and unfinished devices and device components, containers, labeling for regulated products, and all documents that are required to be kept by the regulations, such as device master records and device history records.

Despite the broad inspectional authority over restricted devices, the statute provides that regardless of the device's unrestricted status, certain information is excluded from FDA's inspectional gambit. The kind of information to which FDA does not have access includes financial data, sales data, and pricing data. The new Quality System Regulation, released in 1996, gives the FDA authority to inspect the design area and the qualifications of personnel in all aspects of the product development process.

2.8 A Look at the Future

Reform is inevitable at the FDA. There are signs that Congress will pass the first serious FDA-downsizing federal budget and possibly make its final move on separate FDA reform legislation. Facing serious budgetary cuts, the FDA is looking at alternative methods of operation. Some suggested reforms include:

- Shifting the reviewer force from low-risk device 510(k)s to PMA applications, pre-1976 devices, and device reclassification. The result would be timelier reviews while maintaining scientific rigor.
- Diverting reviewers from lower-risk devices to the more technically complex 510(k) submissions that usually require clinical data. The remaining devices could be farmed out to external reviews or exempted from 510(k) review altogether. Another possibility is self-certification or third-party certification that the devices conform to recognized consensus standards or self-certification by the manufacturer that their devices conform to the FDA's design control requirement.
- Reforming medical device reporting (MDR) management to make greater use of summaries and electronic filing. Thus fewer people would be needed to shuffle paper.
- Reducing the number of routine inspections and focusing on compliance inspections and for-cause (enforcement) inspections.

Not only is the FDA considering these procedural economies, but it is also trying to reengineer the way it does business, in order to afford greater efficiency while retaining a high level of consumer protection.

References

Banta, H. David, "The Regulation of Medical Devices," in *Preventive Medicine*. Volume 19, Number 6, November, 1990.

Basile, Edward, "Overview of Current FDA Requirements for Medical Devices," in *The Medical Device Industry: Science, Technology, and Regulation in a Competitive Environment*. New York: Marcel Dekker, Inc., 1990.

Basile, Edward M. and Alexis J. Prease, "Compiling a Successful PMA Application," in *The Medical Device Industry: Science, Technology, and Regulation in a Competitive Environment*. New York: Marcel Dekker, Inc., 1990.

Bureau of Medical Devices, Office of Small Manufacturers Assistance, *Regulatory Requirements for Marketing a Device*. Washington, DC: U.S. Department of Health and Human Services, 1982.

Center for Devices and Radiological Health, *Device Good Manufacturing Practices Manual*. Washington, DC: U.S. Department of Health and Human Services, 1987.

Dickinson, James G., "In Its Bold New Course, FDA Needs Industry Help." In *Medical Device and Diagnostic Industry*. Volume 19, Number 6, June, 1997.

Food and Drug Administration, *Federal Food, Drug and Cosmetic Act, as Amended January, 1979*. Washington, DC: U.S. Government Printing Office, 1979.

Food and Drug Administration, *Guide to the Inspection of Computerized Systems in Drug Processing*. Washington, DC: Food and Drug Administration, 1983.

Food and Drug Administration, *FDA Policy for the Regulation of Computer Products (Draft)*. Washington, DC: Federal Register, 1987.

Food and Drug Administration, *Software Development Activities*. Washington, DC: Food and Drug Administration, 1987.

Food and Drug Administration, *Medical Devices GMP Guidance for FDA Inspectors*. Washington, DC: Food and Drug Administration, 1987.

Food and Drug Administration, *Reviewer Guidance for Computer-Controlled Medical Devices (Draft)*. Washington, DC: Food and Drug Administration, 1988.

Food and Drug Administration, *Investigational Device Exemptions Manual*. Rockville, MD: Center for Devices and Radiological Health, 1992.

Food and Drug Administration, *Premarket Notification 510(k): Regulatory Requirements for Medical Devices*. Rockville, MD: Center for Devices and Radiological Health, 1992.

Food and Drug Administration, *Premarket Approval (PMA) Manual*. Rockville, MD: Center for Devices and Radiological Health, 1993.

Food and Drug Administration, *Design Control Guidance for Medical Device Manufacturers (Draft)*. Rockville, MD: Center for Devices and Radiological Health, 1996.

Food and Drug Administration, *Do It By Design: An Introduction to Human Factors in Medical Devices*. Draft. Rockville, MD: Center for Devices and Radiological Health, 1996.

Food and Drug Administration, *Quality System Regulation*. Rockville, MD: Department of Health and Human Services, 1996.

Food and Drug Administration, *A New 510(k) Paradigm: Alternate Approaches to Demonstrating Substantial Equivalence in Premarket Notification*. Draft. Rockville, MD: Department of Health and Human Services, 1997.

Fries, Richard C., *Reliable Design of Medical Devices.* New York: Marcel Dekker, Inc., 1997.

Fries, Richard C. et al., "Software Regulation" in *The Medical Device Industry: Science, Technology, and Regulation in a Competitive Environment.* New York: Marcel Dekker, Inc., 1990.

Ginzburg, Harold M., "Protection of Research Subjects in Clinical Research," in *Legal Aspects of Medicine.* New York: Springer-Verlag, 1989.

Gundaker, Walter E., "FDA's Regulatory Program for Medical Devices and Diagnostics," in *The Medical Device Industry: Science, Technology, and Regulation in a Competitive Environment.* New York: Marcel Dekker, Inc., 1990.

Holstein, Howard M., "How to Submit a Successful 510(k)," in *The Medical Device Industry: Science, Technology, and Regulation in a Competitive Environment.* New York: Marcel Dekker, Inc., 1990.

Jorgens III, J. and C. W. Burch, "FDA Regulation of Computerized Medical Devices," *Byte.* Volume 7, 1982.

Jorgens III, J., "Computer Hardware and Software as Medical Devices," *Medical Device and Diagnostic Industry.* May, 1983.

Jorgens III, J. and R. Schneider, "Regulation of Medical Software by the FDA," *Software in Health Care.* April-May, 1985.

Kahan, J. S., "Regulation of Computer Hardware and Software as Medical Devices," *Canadian Computer Law Reporter.* Volume 6, Number 3, January, 1987.

Munsey, Rodney R. and Howard M. Holstein, "FDA/GMP/MDR Inspections: Obligations and Rights," in *The Medical Device Industry: Science, Technology, and Regulation in a Competitive Environment.* New York: Marcel Dekker, Inc., 1990.

Office of Technology Assessment, Federal Policies and the Medical Devices Industry. Washington, DC: U.S. Government Printing Office, 1984.

Sheretz, Robert J. and Stephen A. Streed, "Medical Devices - Significant Risk vs Nonsignificant Risk," in *Journal of the American Medical Association,*

Volume 272, Number 12, September 28, 1994.

Trull, Frankie L. and Barbara A. Rich, "The Animal Testing Issue," in *The Medical Device Industry: Science, Technology, and Regulation in a Competitive Environment*. New York: Marcel Dekker, Inc., 1990.

U. S. Congress, House Committee on Interstate and Foreign Commerce. Medical Devices. Hearings before the Subcommittee on Public Health and the Environment. Octover 23-24, 1973. Serial Numbers 93-61 Washington DC: U.S. Government Printing Office, 1973.

Wholey, Mark H. and Jordan D. Hailer, "An Introduction to the Food and Drug Administration and How It Evaluates New Devices: Establishing Safety and Efficacy," in *CardioVascular and Interventional Radiology*. Volume 18, Number 2, March/April 1995.

Chapter 3

The European Union

The drive toward the creation of a single European economic entity began in 1957 with the signing of the Treaty of Rome. In 1986, the Single European Act established the goal of achieving a single market by 1992 to include 12 member states and approximately 350 million people. Common legislation, the so-called European Directives, were scheduled to cover the entire market. The intention of the European Community (EC) 1992 process was to streamline the approval process for products marketed in the 12 member states. Conceivably, the five member nations of the European Free Trade Association would also recognize the European Directives, even though these nations do not belong to the new common market.

Nearly 300 European Commission Directives have been approved to support implementation of a unified internal market. These directives are not detailed, but rather contain information regarding general *essential requirements*. European regional standards setting bodies are responsible for establishing the voluntary standards, which elaborate on the essential requirements.

The European Union was known as the European Community until the Maastricht Treaty took effect in 1993. Present members include:

Austria
Belgium
Denmark
Finland
France
Germany
Greece
Ireland
Italy
Luxembourg
The Netherlands
Portugal
Spain
Sweden
The United Kingdom.

In 1994, the Agreement on a European Economic Area took effect, adding Iceland, Liechtenstein, and Norway to the single market, although they did not join the European Union. These 18 countries comprise a market approximately the size of the North American Free Trade Agreement.

Standards serve as an essential component in assuring the complete freedom of trade in merchandise across national borders. Standard bodies in the member states are obliged to adopt European standards and withdraw conflicting national standards. Harmonized, European-wide standards in key product sectors are now replacing the thousands of differing national standards that existed within member states. Today, the European standardization system has almost 5,000 standards and produces approximately five new standards per working day.

3.1 European Directives

In the period up to 1992, and subsequently, the European Parliament has enacted a series of measures intended to put the single market into practice. Some of these directives have been aimed at removing barriers of a purely customs/excise nature, while others have concentrated on transport arrangements to ensure the free movement of goods. A series of directives, produced under the heading of "New Approach Directives," are intended to provide controls on product design, with the principal objective being to provide a level playing field for product safety requirements across the European Union.

The primary function of these directives is to ensure that products are sufficiently well designed and built to be fit for the purpose for which they are sold, and that reasonable precautions are taken to protect the user against injury while the product is being used. Recent directives have included provisions for medical devices and electromagnetic compatibility.

In the past, the European Union relied on harmonized legislation to enforce common production standards, without reference to voluntary standards or a marking system. Under this old approach, directives contained such a high degree of detail on the technical specifications of products, it sometimes required a decade or more to complete the technical work.

Now, the new approach directives specify only the *essential requirements* to be met by products and that the technical specifications governing the production and marketing of products meeting the essential requirements be laid down by the relevant European standardization bodies.

3.2 European Standardization Bodies

Under this approach, the European Commission mandated that the private sector be responsible for development of European technical standards. Three regional standards organizations were assigned the task:

- The European Committee for Standardization (CEN),
- The European Committee for Electrotechnical Standardization (CENELEC),
- The European Telecommunications Standards Institute (ETSI).

CEN, CENELEC, and ETSI constitute a European forum for standardization that organizes participation of all parties concerned in the development and standardization programs. These parties include national government authorities, the Commission of European Communities (commonly known as the European Commission) the European Free Trade Association, public bodies, manufacturers, trade unions, users, and consumers. These parties come together in hundreds of technical groups to prepare European standards through procedures that guarantee respect for the principles of openness and transparency, consensus, national commitment, technical coherence at the national and European level, and correct integration with other international work. Consequently, the development of standards within the national bodies of the European Union essentially ceased and work was transferred into the European standards organizations.

Many multinational manufacturers have globalized their product development efforts. Until recently, they have regarded the FDA as the agency with the most experience in regulating medical devices. The EC 1992 process splits the burden of stringent regulation between the United States and the European Commission. Many of these multinational manufacturers have grown accustomed to dealing with U.S. bureaucracy, but now will have to work also with the incipient EC bureaucracy in Brussels. Unraveling the complex European process is extremely difficult. Change is rapid and what is established as fact this week, may be overturned or obsolete next week.

These complex changes and the bureaucracy being created in Brussels are being driven by seven major groups of organizations. The groups consist of the following:

- the European Commission,
- standing committees,
- standards organizations,
- Notified Bodies,
- Board of Health,
- Ethical Committee.

The European Commission, one of the three major branches of the European government, is the primary force of change. Another branch, the European Parliament, debates the directives proposed by the Commission. The third branch, the Court of Justice, will adjudicate any differences that arise between parties within the European Community.

The three medical device directives create standing committees, which after the European Commission, constitute the second major force behind the European regulatory changes. Each directive creates two committees, which could be combined into one major standing committee that would address differences between essential requirements outlined in all the directives and international or European normalized standards. The second standing committee, which might vary depending upon the directive, would address specific issues relevant to that directive. What have been termed *competent authorities*, namely the boards of health of the 12 member states, constitute another major force behind these changes.

Notified Bodies compose yet another force for change. In reality, these are the test houses that are designated by individual member states' board of health. Some states may have more than one test house, and smaller countries may have none. Those member states that do not designate a Notified Body will delegate their medical device issues to member states that have larger and more resourceful boards of health and Notified Bodies.

Ethical committees at EC medical institutions also play an important role in evaluating investigational devices. Many European teaching institutions already have ethics committees properly constituted and duly functioning. Many non-teaching institutions, however, do not have such committees and will be required to form them.

These organizational forces are, and will remain, highly interactive. Many institutions are working diligently at what they perceive to be their mandate. From the United States perspective, the European process is producing a great deal of activity and, in some cases, significant action. It is clear that many organizations are working to change the legislative and regulatory environment for medical devices in Europe.

3.3 European Standards Development Process

Through their standardization work, CEN, CENELEC, and ETSI aim to remove any differences of a technical nature, either between the national standards of the member states or between measures applied at the national level to certify conformity, that could give rise to technical barriers to trade. In the areas of technology, European Standards are prepared following specific requests from the European Commission and the European Free Trade Association.

3.3.1 New Work

The Dresden Agreement, between CENELEC and IEC, gives IEC the "Right of First Refusal" for work proposed in CENELEC. According to the Vienna Agreement, CEN must determine whether it is possible to give preference to ISO to develop a new project, noting that a completed standards project must be available within specific timeframes. ISO has three months to respond to any such request received from CEN. CEN must also consider its various procedural options and, if the CEN technical committee decides to propose the work item to ISO, work will commence following the normal procedures in one of the following scenarios:

- new work falling within the scope of an existing ISO technical committee and subcommittee

technical committee and subcommittee
- new work requiring an extension of the scope of an existing ISO technical committee
- new work proposed that falls into a field(s) not yet covered in ISO.

3.3.2 Development

Most European Standards not taken from one of the international standardization organizations are developed in working groups reporting to technical committees or subcommittees of the regional European standards organizations. Access to this process by U.S. interests has been acquired in four ways:

- Under the Vienna and Dresden Agreements, the relevant ISO or IEC/RCs or SCs can appoint a representative, preferably no more than two, to the parallel European activity, including working groups
- ANSI can officially request that an American be allowed to attend a working group meeting(s) as an observer
- Interests with representatives in Europe can become members of a European country's delegation and participate directly
- Informal agreements between U.S. interests and their counterparts in CEN or CENELEC working groups allow participation.

3.3.3 Public Enquiry

Public enquiry is a six month time period during which the European members can offer national body comments. This is not a voting stage. Under the Vienna and Dresden Agreements, CEN and CENELEC have agreed to accept comments on preliminary European Standards (prEN) and preliminary Harmonized Documents (prHD) from ISO and IEC member bodies. ANSI, as the U.S. member body, announces availability of all prENs and prHDs in ANSI's Standards Action and via their site on the world wide web. Enquiry drafts can be purchased from ANSI's Customer Services Department and comments submitted via staff in ANSI's Standards Facilitation Department. U.S. comments are sent to the offices of the respective Central Secretariat in Brussels and are referred to the applicable technical committee for response.

Replies to U.S. comments are received in due course by ANSI and referred back to the originator in the United States.

3.3.4 Formal Vote

CEN, CENELEC, and ETSI are populated at the formal vote stage by member countries, not by individuals. National delegations have weighted votes, applied for by the national body and confirmed by the General Assemblies of the respective organizations.

The United States, as a non-member nation, does not have a vote. If ANSI were to be a member and have a vote in these organizations, the United States would be obligated by the respective Operating Procedures to adopt and implement approved ENs at the national level and to withdraw any conflicting national standard. U.S. interests have indicated that they are unwilling to accept as a matter of course the outright adoption as national standards of all documents developed and approved by the European standardization bodies.

Further, within the European regional bodies, the U.S. would have only one vote, even if weighted to some extent. Through ANSI, the U.S. has considerably more options in lining up support for issues arising under the purview of the ISO and IEC. In the international arena, even though it is still one country - one vote, ANSI can call upon allies in the Pan American Standards Commission (COPANT) and the Pacific Area Standards Congress (PASC) for supporting votes from outside Europe.

ANSI does, however, publish notice of the two month formal vote stage in Standards Action. The formal vote documents, which in most cases become the approved European Standard, are available for sale through ANSI's Customer Services Department.

3.3.5 Publication

ETSI publishes its final documents following approval by its constituents. Member countries are responsible for publishing European Standards approved by CEN and CENELEC. ANSI obtains and sells ENs upon request.

3.4 Other European Standards Considerations

3.4.1 Primary Questionnaire Procedure

In order to test the market need for a standard, a Primary Questionnaire (PQ) has been developed. The PQ procedure permits CEN or CENELEC to determine whether enough interest exists in harmonization on the subject proposed, the existing degree of national harmonization on the reference document in question, and whether the document would be acceptable as an EN, HD, or ENV. The PQ procedure serves the same purpose as the six-month enquiry procedure and concerns entirely new documents being offered to CEN or CENELEC.

3.4.2 Dual Regional and International Work

If European regional activities are already underway and the international community attempts to begin a similar activity, the Europeans may resist the suggestion for a new international committee. As an alternative, the European regional body may suggest that they will "fast-track" their work into ISO or IEC, as appropriate, at the enquiry stage (DIS or CDV, respectively), thereby providing non-Europeans with an opportunity to cast a national body position during the fast-track DIS or CDV ballot. The problem, however, is that comments will be forwarded back to the regional body for response. This scenario provides relatively little input for non-Europeans to participate in the development of the project.

When faced with this situation, the affected U.S. industry sector, normally working through a trade association or professional society and via ANSI, must actively persuade other non-European countries of the necessity of doing the work in an international organization like ISO or IEC. The United States should be extremely confident that it has the required number of allies guaranteed to support the formation of a new ISO or IEC TC or SC prior to ANSI or USNC submission of the proposal for a new area of technical work.

3.4.3 Parallel Voting

According to the Lugano Agreement, only DIS (Draft International Standards) were processed for parallel voting both within IEC and CENELEC. Now with the approval of the Dresden Agreement, IEC working drafts will also be sent to CENELEC for parallel review and comment. This procedure makes it more likely that the draft standard will be accepted not only internationally, but also as an identical European standard.

The Vienna Agreement also provides for parallel voting at the DIS and FDIS (Final Draft International Standard) level. If mutual agreement is reached, the International Standard (IS) and EN would be published concurrently. The submitting organization is responsible for responding to comments during voting.

3.4.4 Unique Acceptance Procedure

The Unique Acceptance Procedure (UAP) may be applied in any type of document, whatever its origin, in order to achieve rapid approval of an EN or HD, if it is reasonable to suppose that the document is acceptable at the European level. For a reference document, the UAP combines the questionnaire procedure and the formal vote.

If CEN or CENELEC modify an international standard, ISO or IEC must either agree to incorporate the changes into a new international standard, or the regional bodies shall adopt the revised text as a regional, but not international, standard.

3.5 Conformity Assessment and Testing

The European Commission has supported its program of directives for the elimination of technical barriers to trade with a selection of harmonized conformity modules and with the use of a harmonized European mark, the CE mark.

The purpose of the directives is not to ban any products from the European Union single market, unless the product is very poorly made or is unsafe. For most reputable manufacturers, complying with the essential protection requirements of the directives is not particularly onerous and companies that have always taken a responsible attitude to the performance and design of their products will have few problems complying with the directives.

3.5.1 The CE Mark

CE marking does not indicate conformity to a standard, but rather indicates conformity to the legal requirements of EU directives. Many of the EU directives require manufacturers to have a Certified Quality System conforming to ISO 9000 in operation and to use the assistance of a Notified Body in order that the manufacturer can legitimately apply the CE marking to their product.

As there may be difficulties in the administrative requirements, a new way of working for some manufacturers and suppliers, particularly small businesses, may be required. Manufacturers may well find it cost effective to seek outside help in the early stages of complying with the directives, in order to save time and prevent expensive mistakes. However, it is important to be aware that it is rarely necessary to commit to an expensive program of testing and certification. Unless the directives applying to the product specifically require the involvement of a third party for product approval or quality system assessment, the manufacturer can affix the mark without having to involve test house, consultant or anyone else.

The CE mark (Figure 3-1) must be affixed to the product, its instructional manual, or its packaging. It must be at least 5 mm high. It is not intended to be a mark of quality. Rather, it is intended to indicate to the authorities responsible for enforcing the directives that the product's manufacturer claims compliance with the directives that apply to the product.

The act of fixing the mark to the product, and signing the Declaration of Conformity, constitutes a declaration by the manufacturer that the product meets the requirements of all the directives that apply to it. The onus is very much on the manufacturer to take responsibility for this actually being true. Marking a product which is not fully in accordance with the requirements of the applicable directives is an offense in its own right, and would also contravene related consumer safety and trade description legislation.

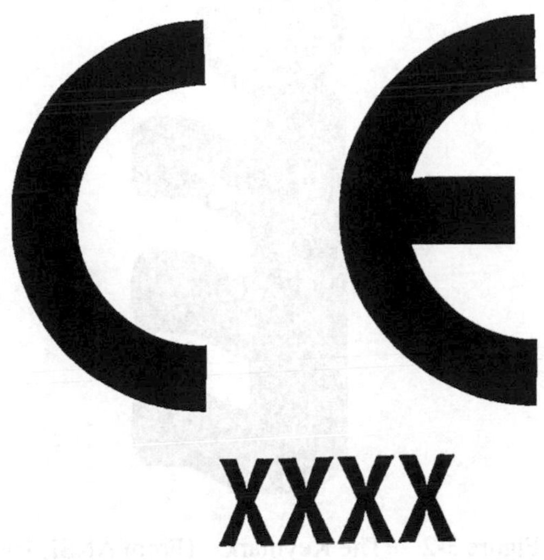

Figure 3-1 The CE Mark. (From Fries, 1997)

3.5.2 The Keymark

The purpose of the "Keymark" (Figure 3-2) is to make available to European industry a voluntary harmonized service that provides for the independent third-party testing of products and to ensure compliance with the requirements of the relevant European Standards developed by CEN or CENELEC. The Keymark also requires confirmation of the manufacturer's quality management system. To ensure that quality is maintained, both the manufacturer and the product will be subject to regular assessment.

Contrary to the mandatory "CE" mark, use of the Keymark is voluntary. The Keymark may replace many, if not all, of the numerous national certification marks for products which are sold throughout Europe. It is expected that there will be a reduction in costs related to certification, which will impact the consumer at another level.

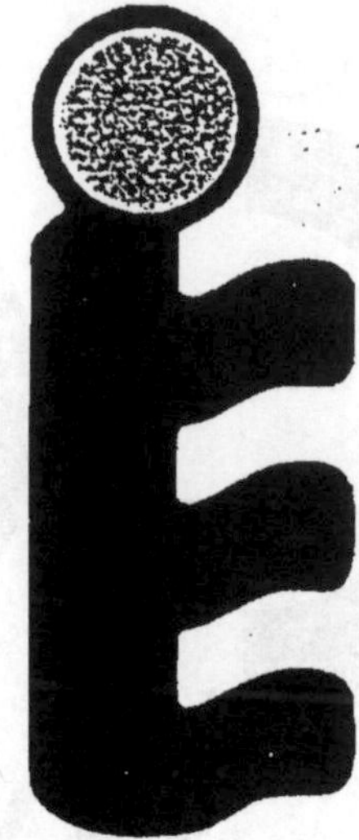

Figure 3-2 The Keymark. (From ANSI, 1996)

The U.S. will monitor use of the mark to ensure that it does not become de facto mandatory as, for example, in procurements.

3.6 European Organization for Testing and Certification

The European Organization for Testing and Certification (EOTC) was established in April, 1990 by the European Commission, the European Free Trade Association, and the European Standards Bodies. Articles of Association were signed by the 22 founding members on December 3, 1992, and the EOTC attained a legal status under Belgian law in April, 1993. EOTC members are testing and calibration laboratories with help and input from certification bodies, manufacturers, and trade associations. The customer base of EOTC is composed of suppliers, manufacturers, purchasers, and users of goods and services and all those who benefit from the development of mutual recognition in any sector.

The EOTC acts as a focal point for conformity assessment issues in Europe, but does not itself test or certify products or services. Testing is performed by recognized Agreement Groups consisting of test laboratories or certification bodies.

3.7 The NVCASE Program

The United States has been actively negotiating with the EU to develop a Mutual Recognition Agreement (MRA) concerning the acceptance of mutual conformity assessment programs. The National Institute of Standards and Technology (NIST), through its Office of Standards Services, has established a fee-for-service, voluntary program entitled the National Voluntary Conformity Assessment System Evaluation (NVCASE). It evaluates and recognizes organizations which support conformity assessment activities.

The United States has proposed that NVCASE recognition be one means of acceptance by the EU, of U.S. bodies as equivalent to EU notified bodies, to approve products for entry to the EU marketplace. The National Voluntary Conformity Assessment Evaluation Program (NVCAEP) includes activities related to laboratory testing, product certification, and quality system registration. After NVCASE evaluation, NIST provides recognition to qualified United States organizations that effectively demonstrate conformance with established criteria. The ultimate goal is to help United States manufacturers satisfy applicable product requirements mandated by other countries through conformity assessment procedures conducted in this country prior to export.

Conformity assessment activities may be considered to be conducted at three levels:

- the conformity level, such as product testing, product certification, and quality system registration
- the accreditation level, such as the actions of accreditors of bodies operating at the conformity level
- the recognition of accreditors.

NVCASE recognition provides other governments with a basis for having confidence in the fact that qualifying United States conformity assessment bodies are competent, and facilitates the acceptance of United States products in foreign regulated markets based on U.S. conformity assessment results.

References

American National Standards Institute (ANSI), *American Access to the European Standardization Process.* New York: American National Standards Institute, 1996.

CEN/CENELAC, *Directory of the European Standardization Requirements for Health Care Informatics and Programme for the Development of Standards.* Brussels, Belgium: European Committee for Standardization, 1992

CEN/CENELAC, *EN 46001*. Brussels, Belgium: European Committee for Standardization, 1995

CEN/CENELAC, *EN 46002*. Brussels, Belgium: European Committee for Standardization, 1995

Department of Trade and Industry, *Guide to Software Quality Management System Construction and Certification Using EN 29001*. London: DISC TickIT Office, 1987.

Donaldson, John, "U.S. Companies Gear Up for ISO 14001 Certification," in *In Tech.* Volume 43, Number 5, May, 1996.

Fries, Richard C., *Reliable Medical Device Design.* New York: Marcel Dekker, Inc., 1997.

International Standard Organization, *Quality Management and Quality Assurance Standards - Part 3: Guidelines for the Application of ISO 9001 to the Development, Supply and Maintenance of Software*. Geneva, Switzerland: International Organization for Standardization, 1991.

Meeldijk, Victor, *Electronic Components: Selection and Application Guidelines.* New York: John Wiley & Sons, Inc., 1996.

Schaefer, Jack, "Europe 1992: Organizational Structure, Administrative Procedures, and Proposed Regulations," in *Medical Design and Material.* Volume 1, Number 2, February, 1991.

Shaw, Roger, "Safety Critical Software and Current Standards Initiatives," in *Computer Methods and Programs in Biomedicine*. Volume 44, Number 1, July, 1994.

Tabor, Tom and Ira Feldman, *ISO 14000: A Guide to the New Environmental Management Standards*. Milwaukee, WI: The American Society for Quality Control, 1996.

Working Group #4, *Draft of Proposed Regulatory Requirements for Medical Devices Sold in Canada*. Ottawa, Ontario Canada: Environmental Heal Directorate, 1995.

Chapter 4

The Global Harmonization Task Force

The Global Harmonization Task Force was formed in September, 1992 with the goal of facilitating the mutual recognition of quality system approvals relating to medical devices. The Task Force was sponsored by the European Commission and is made up of delegates from industry and government in Australia, Canada, Europe, Japan, Mexico, and the United States. At its first meeting, the Task Force set as its goal the assurance that the internationally recognized ISO 9000 series of quality system standards was interpreted in each country's law in an equivalent way.

To date, many countries have welcomed the comments and advice of the Task Force without the existence of a formal structure or formal obligations. The comments of the Task Force on national draft regulations have been considered in detail by the countries concerned with regard to current regulations. Nevertheless, there is a need for more discussion on how to give greater political impact to the Task Force's documents.

4.1 Objectives of the Task Force

The Global Harmonization Task Force has taken on the following objectives:

- to examine differing supplementary requirements to ISO 9001/9002 and agree or propose textual changes to bring them into alignment.
- to examine the need for new documents or programs that would help in the uniform application and inspection of quality systems and identify the steps needed to create them.

Three new study groups were initially formed to help the task force in meeting its objectives. The responsibilities of each group were:

Study Group I: Comparison of Regulatory Schemes

> The Group will consider regulatory systems in the United States, Canada, Japan, and the European Community for selection of medical devices. The purpose will be to evaluate and compare all aspects of product approval processes.

Study Group II: Harmonization of the FDA/GMP and EN 46001

> The Group will work toward aligning the United States' GMP system and Europe's prEN 46001.

Study Group III: Guidance Documents

> The Group will aim to harmonize all existing or draft guidance quality system documents into one general guidance document for manufacturers and inspectors of medical devices. Appendices may have to be harmonized for specific issues, such as sterilization, software, and clean rooms.

The Global Harmonization Task Force attempts to fulfill its goals by taking on the following tasks:

- examining the supplementary requirements to ISO 9001 and 9002 and agreeing or proposing textual changes to bring them into alignment
- examining available or draft guidance documents to quality system standards for use by manufacturers and or inspectors, and agreeing or proposing steps to bring them into alignment
- examining available or draft documents addressing issues related to quality systems and agreeing or proposing steps to bring them

into alignment

- examining the need for new documents or programs that would facilitate the uniform application and inspection of quality systems and identifying the steps needed to bring them into existence
- recognizing the need for and developing the procedure for the establishment of an internationally harmonized nomenclature system for medical devices.

4.2 Philosophy of the Task Force

Work on a global vigilance system for medical devices will be based on the philosophy and structure of the European system. While national quality systems differ, there are areas of common ground where harmonization could be achieved. Harmonization of requirements is regarded as a feasible first step toward the ultimate goal of mutual recognition.

4.3 Current Activities

The Global Harmonization Task Force currently has four active study groups:

Study Group 1	Regulatory Systems
Study Group 2	Post-Market Surveillance
Study Group 3	Quality Systems
Study Group 4	Quality Systems Auditing

Working Group 1 is involved with examining medical device regulatory systems in use in the major trading countries/regions to identify features of those systems which have a common basis, but different applications, identifying features peculiar to individual systems, which may present obstacles to uniform regulation, making proposals to the Task Force for harmonization activities relating to these features, and suggesting priorities.

Working Group 2 is involved with working on the harmonization of requirements for reporting adverse events, device nomenclature, and requirements for exchange of regulatory data.

Working Group 3 is involved with issuing guidance on the implementation of quality systems, and working on guidance for design control and process validation.

Working Group 4 is involved with developing guidance on the auditing of quality systems for the design and manufacture of medical devices.

References

"Global Harmonisation Task Force sets its agenda," in *Clinica World Medical Device And Diagnostic News.* February 17, 1993

"Global harmonisation of medical device regulation," in *Clinica World Medical Device And Diagnostic News.* October 6, 1993.

"Differences in quality systems reviewed," in *Clinica World Medical Device And Diagnostic News.* November 24, 1993.

"Stepwise approach to global harmonisation," in *Clinica World Medical Device And Diagnostic News.* July 10, 1995.

"Harmonisation of US device-approved regulations," in *Clinica World Medical Device And Diagnostic News.* July 31, 1995.

"European vigilance to be model for global system," in *Clinica World Medical Device And Diagnostic News.* March 18, 1996.

"Changes ahead for Global Harmonisation Task Force," in *Clinica World Medical Device And Diagnostic News.* October 21, 1996.

"Harmonization efforts will bring more data to FDA," in *Devices & Diagnostics Letter.* Volume 23, Number 43, November 8, 1996.

"U.S. and EU industry split over new ISO device committee," in *Europe Drug & Device Report.* Volume 4, Number 16, August 8, 1994.

"Harmonizing quality system auditing stresses interest conflicts," in *Europe Drug & Device Report.* Volume 6, Number 9, April 29, 1996.

"International device harmonization a double-edged sword," in *Europe Drug & Device Report.* Volume 6, Number 23, December 9, 1996.

Chapter 5

The Special Case for Software

Since the time software was first used in a medical device, it has always been treated as a special entity by standards and regulatory agencies. Because it was something that could not be touched, it has been treated as if it were some alien life form come to test the resolve of any standards or regulatory professional. In part, this has come from an apparent lack of understanding of what software really is and how it performs, thus leading to over regulation.

Software, in and of itself, does not fail. Software is merely a set of instructions which the computing device will follow exactly as it is written. Software failures are significantly different from those of hardware components. There are four basic causes of software failures: specification errors, design errors, typographical errors, and omissions of symbols. Thus, many standards and regulations address the process of developing the software, dealing primarily with "best practices." Requirements are drawn from this set of best practices.

5.1 Software as a Technology

Software is a set of instructions that, when executed, allows the desired function and performance of a program to be realized. The term software includes 1) data structures that enable the program to manipulate information and 2) documentation that describes the operation and the use of the program.

Software differs from hardware in several important respects. Software is a logical rather than a physical element. Software is developed rather than manufactured in the classical sense. Software does not wear out as hardware does. Software costs are concentrated in engineering.

Software quality is a primary concern of software developers. Poor quality is costly, damages the company's reputation, reduces its market share, and puts the manufacturer at risk for liability. Quality attributes that are important characteristics of any software product include:

- usefulness - satisfying user needs
- preciseness - clearly written and easily understood
- efficiency - doing what it has been designed to do
- cost effectiveness - the greatest benefit for the least cost
- reliability - assuring performance to specification, without failure, under stated conditions, for a specified period of time.

The subject of software quality is the subject of many standards and regulations.

5.2 Domestic Software Regulation

In the United States, the FDA is responsible for assuring the device utilizing software or the software as a device is safe and effective for its intended use. The Quality System Regulation addresses software as part of the design phase. The FDA has produced several drafts of reviewer guidelines, auditor guidelines, software policy, and GMP regulations addressing both device and process software. In addition, guidelines for FDA reviewers as well as training programs for inspectors and reviewers have been prepared.

5.2.1 The FDA and Software

The subject of software in and as a medical device has become an important topic for the FDA. This interest began in 1985 when software in a radiation treatment therapy device is alleged to have resulted in a lethal overdose. The FDA then analyzed recalls by fiscal year to determine how many were caused by software problems. In 1985, for example, 20% of all neurology device recalls were attributable to software problems, while 8% of cardiovascular problems had the same cause. This type of analysis, along with the results of various corporate inspections, led the FDA to conclude that some type of regulation was required.

Since there are many types of software in use in the medical arena, the problem of the best way to regulate it has become an issue for the FDA. Discussions have centered around what type of software is a medical device, the type of regulation required for such software, and what could be inspected under current regulations. Agency concerns fall into three major categories: medical device software, software used in manufacturing, and software information systems used for clinical decision making.

For medical device software, the FDA is responsible for ensuring that the device utilizing the software is safe and effective. It only takes a few serious injuries or deaths to sensitize the agency to a particular product or generic component that deserves attention. The Agency's review of medical device reporting (MDR) incidents and analysis of product recalls has convinced the Agency that software is a factor contributing to practical problems within devices.

When software is used during manufacturing, the FDA is concerned with whether or not the software controlling a tool or automatic tester is performing as expected. The FDA's perceptions are rooted in experiences with GMP inspections of pharmaceutical manufacturers, where computers are heavily depended upon for control of manufacturing processes. Although there are few incidents of device or manufacturing problems traceable to flaws in manufacturing software, GMP inspections have focused intensively on validation of software programs used in industry for control of manufacturing operations.

With regard to stand-alone software used to aid clinical decision making, the FDA is concerned with hypothetical problems rather than extensive records of adverse incidents. While most commercially available health care information systems replace manual systems that had a far higher potential for errors, the FDA believes that regulations should apply to the kinds of systems that may influence clinical treatment or diagnoses. FDA has observed academic work of "expert systems" used by medical professionals and is concerned that such systems may be commercialized without sufficient controls.

A draft of a software policy was issued in September, 1987. The policy was a general statement of FDA thinking, including the definition of a medical device, establishment of a three class system for regulation of software, and a list of exemptions from the regulations. The draft is very general and leaves much room for personal interpretation. The draft does not address GMP issues nor the status of software as an inspectable commodity. The draft was revised in 1989, but did little to clear up the above issues. To date, a final policy has not been published.

The FDA has published guidelines for developing quality software, the requirements for product approval submissions (510k) and the inspection of software controlled test fixtures as a part of GMP inspections. Recent documents address software validation and the use of off-the-shelf software packages in medical devices. They have also conducted training courses for their inspectors and submission reviewers on the subject of software and computer basics.

5.2.2 Software Classification

When a computer product is a component, part, or accessory of a product recognized as a medical device in its own right, the computer component is regulated according to the requirements for the parent device unless the component of the device is separately classified. Computer products that are medical devices and not components, parts or accessories of other products that are themselves medical devices are subject to one of three degrees of regulatory control depending on their characteristics. These products are regulated with the least degree of control necessary to provide reasonable assurance of safety and effectiveness. Computer products that are substantially equivalent to a device previously classified will be regulated to the same degree as the equivalent device. Those devices that are not substantially equivalent to a preamendment device or that are substantially equivalent to a Class III device are regulated as Class III devices.

Software classification, as listed in the FDA draft policy of 1987, follows a similar pattern to devices. Medical software is divided into three classes with regulatory requirements specific to each:

Class I software is subject to the FFD&C Act's general controls relating to such matters as misbranding, registration of manufacturers, record keeping, and good manufacturing practices. An example of Class I software would be a program that calculates the composition of infant formula.

Class II software is that for which general controls are insufficient to provide reasonable assurance of safety and effectiveness and for which performance standards can provide assurance. This is exemplified by a computer program designed to produce radiation therapy treatment plans.

Class III software is that for which insufficient information exists to ensure that general controls and performance standards will provide reasonable assurance of safety and effectiveness. Generally, these devices are represented to be life-sustaining or life-supporting and may be intended for a use that is of substantial importance in preventing impairment to health. They may be implanted in the body or present a potential unreasonable risk of illness or injury. A program that measures glucose levels and calculates and dispenses insulin based upon those calculations without physician intervention would be a Class III device.

5.3 Domestic Software Standards

There are a myriad of software standards to assist the developer in designing and documenting their program. IEEE standards cover documentation through all phases of design. Military standards describe how software is to be designed and developed for military use. There are also standards on software quality and reliability to assist developers in preparing a quality program. The international community has produced standards, primarily dealing with software safety. In each case, the standard is a voluntary document that has been developed to provide guidelines for designing, developing, testing, and documenting a software program.

5.4 International Software Regulations

The Medical Device Directives address software in their definition of a medical device:

> "any instrument, appliance, apparatus, material or other article, whether used alone or in combination, including the software necessary for its proper application, intended by the manufacturer to be used for human beings for the purpose of:

> diagnosis, prevention, monitoring, treatment or alleviation of disease;
>
> diagnosis, monitoring, alleviation of or compensation for an injury or handicap;
>
> investigation, replacement or modification of the anatomy or of a physiological process;
>
> control of conception;
>
> and which does not achieve its principal intended action in or on the human body by pharmacological, immunological or metabolic means, but which may be assisted in its function by such means."

The software definition will probably be given further interpretation, but is currently interpreted to mean that 1) software intended to control the function of a device is a medical device, 2) software for patient records or other administrative purposes is not a device, 3) software which is built into a device, e.g., software in an electrocardiographic monitor used to drive a display, is clearly an integral part of the medical device, 4) a software update sold by the manufacturer, or a variation sold by a software house, is a medical device in its own right.

5.5 International Software Standards

Several software standards activities are currently underway. They include ISO and IEC standards, the TickIT program, and the Software Quality System Registration Program.

5.5.1 ISO and IEC Standards

ISO 9001 addresses software as part of the design process. ISO 9000-3 specifically addresses software issues in detail, with reference to ISO 9001. Several other ISO and IEC standards address software issues, primarily from the risk management and safety viewpoint. Software issues are also addressed in the application of the ISO 9001 standard to medical devices.

5.5.2 The TickIT Program

The TickIT project came from two studies commissioned by the Department of Trade and Industry (DTI) which showed that the cost of poor quality in software in the United Kingdom was very considerable and that quality system certification was desired by the market. The studies undertook extensive research into the respective subjects and included a broad consultative process with users, suppliers, in-house developers, and purchasers with the primary task being to identify options for harmonization. The reports made a number of significant recommendations, including:

- all Quality Management System standards in common use were generically very similar
- the best harmonization route was through ISO 9001
- action was required to improve market confidence in third party certifications of Quality Management Systems
- there was an urgent need to establish an accredited certification body or bodies for the software sector.

These principal recommendations were accepted by the DTI and further work was commissioned with the British Computer Society (BCS) to set up an acceptable means to gain accredited certification of Quality Management Systems by auditors with necessary expertise. Draft guidance material for an acceptable certification scheme was developed. The onward development from this draft material has become known as the TickIT project.

TickIT is principally a certification scheme, but this is not its primary purpose. The main objectives are to stimulate developers to think about what quality really is and how it may be achieved. Unless certification is purely a by-product of these more fundamental aims, much of the effort will be wasted. To stimulate thinking, TickIT includes some quality themes that give direction to the setting up of a Quality Management System (QMS) and the context of certification.

Generally, TickIT certification applies to Information Technology (IT) systems where software development forms a significant or critical part of the system. The main focus of TickIT is software development because this is the component that gives an information system its power and flexibility. It is also the source of many of the problems.

5.5.3 The Software Quality System Registration Program

The Software Quality System Registration Committee was established in 1992. The Committee's charter was to determine whether a program should be created in the U.S. for ISO 9001 registration of software design, production and supply. A comparable program, TickIT, had been operational in the United Kingdom for over one year and was gaining European acceptance. To ensure mutual recognition and to leverage the experience of the worldwide software industry, the Software Quality System Registration (SQSR) program preserves ISO 9001 as the sole source for requirements and ISO 9000-3 as a source of official guidance for software registrants.

The SQSR program is designed for ISO 9001 registration of suppliers who design and develop software as a significant or crucial element in the products they offer. The SQSR program addresses the unique requirements of software engineering and provides a credible technical basis to allow the Registrar Accreditation Board (RAB) to extend its current programs for accrediting ISO 9000 registrars, certifying auditors, and accrediting specific courses and course providers.

The program is intended to ensure that ISO registration is an effective, enduring indicator of a software supplier's capability. The effectiveness of the SQSR program is based on three factors: mutual recognition, guidance, and an administrative infrastructure tailored to the U.S. marketplace.

5.6 The Move Toward One Software Standard

A task force has been established, with the author as chair, under the auspices of the Association for the Advancement of Medical Instrumentation (AAMI), to address the issue of whether one international software standard could be used for meeting both regulatory and certification needs.

The discussion began with a group consisting of the FDA, AAMI, the Health Industry Manufacturers Association (HIMA), the National Electrical Manufacturers Association (NEMA), Underwriters Laboratory, and industry representatives. FDA expressed the possibility of moving the review of product submissions to a third party and the desire to have one standard, covering both stand-alone and embedded software, that met the submission requirements of the FDA and would be easy for third parties to use for certification. Third parties expressed an interest in having a more detailed standard - one indicating detailed steps that they could follow in the certification process. The group also felt the current IEC 601-1-4 standard did not fully address the requirements for stand-alone software, and therefore they should be included in the new standard.

A survey was conducted to determine what standards software manufacturers were currently using in developing and certifying their software. The results of the survey indicated three standards were most frequently used:

- ISO 9000-3
- IEC 601-1-4
- IEEE Software Standards

The first meeting of the task force took place in March, 1997, in Washington, DC. The conclusions of the meeting were:

- developing one software standard was a good idea
- the standard should be used for regulatory certification
- the standard should be general rather than detailed, because of the many types of software in the marketplace
- the standard should reference the most currently used standards
- the standard should be developed by a joint IEC/ISO technical committee
- the chair should prepare a draft proposal and draft standard for review by the task force prior to submission to the technical committee.

As of this writing, the draft proposal and draft standard are being reviewed. The next meeting of the task force is scheduled for September, 1997 to finalize the proposal and draft for submission to IEC and ISO.

References

Food and Drug Administration, *FDA Policy for the Regulation of Computer Products.* Washington D.C.: Food and Drug Administration, 1987.

Fries, Richard C., George T. Willingmyre, Dee Simons, and Robert T. Schwartz, "Software Regulation." In *The Medical Device Industry: Science, Technology, and Regulation in a Competitive Environment.* New York: Marcel Dekker, Inc., 1990.

Fries, Richard C., *Reliable Design of Medical Devices.* New York: Marcel Dekker, Inc., 1997.

Jorgens, Joseph III, "Computer Hardware and Software as Medical Devices," in *Medical Device and Diagnostic Industry.* May, 1983.

Pressman, R.S., *Software Engineering.* New York: McGraw-Hill, 1987.

Section 2

Quality Systems

Chapter 6

The ISO 9000 Series of Standards

The ISO 9000 standards are a series of internationally accepted standards which specify a quality management system. They judge how well a business is run in delivering a consistent quality product. They deal with all aspects of a business and how controls are managed and improved. They describe a basic set of elements by which an organization can develop and implement a quality management system. Registration to the series of standards is accomplished through a third party audit, by a notified body, which must be approved by an international certification organization. Some examples of notified bodies are British Standards Institute (BSI), Lloyds, and Technischer Überwachungs Verein (TÜV). Registration to these standards ensures an organization, and those that do business with them, of an operating quality management system.

The standards are important externally for several reasons. First, they serve as a benchmark for quality performance. Second, the European Community has adopted them as a quality standard. Third, major customers may require certification to one of the ISO 9000 standards as a requirement to conduct business. Fourth, certification may be required in order to process sales in Europe.

The standards are important internally for several reasons.

Certification establishes a quality system and employee understanding of quality systems. Certification creates active employee participation in establishing the quality system. Certification helps maintain quality improvement gains. Certification places the company on a level playing field with the competition.

6.1 Origin of the ISO 9000 Standards

In 1979, Technical Committee 176 was formed as part of the International Organization for Standardization (ISO) in response to a formal proposal by the British Standard Institute. The committee began work on a unified quality standard using the British standard BS 5750 and the Canadian standard CSA Z299 as the primary inputs. The committee first published the ISO 9000 series of standards in 1987. The standards were revised in 1994.

The ISO 9000 standards enjoyed an unusually wide and early acceptance in Europe and across the world. The European Community has adopted ISO 9000 quality standards. These countries recognize either the ISO 9000 series of EN 29000 under the European norm system for quality system certification.

The impetus for common standards in Europe is driven by the need to normalize individual country standards in favor of international standards. The European Free Trade Association (EFTA) and a total of more than 50 countries, including Japan and the United States have adopted the ISO 9000 series of standards.

The United States representative within ISO is the American National Standards Institute (ANSI). Within the United States, the Department of Defense (DOD) and many major corporations have embraced the ISO 9000 series as the standard their supplier's quality system must meet. In thirty-two countries, including the United States, the customer will recognize that a supplier's quality system meets the requirements of the appropriate ISO 9000 standard if that customer is registered by a third-party accredited registrar.

6.2 The Role of the ISO 9000 Standards

The ISO 9000 series standards have two primary roles. The series provide guidance for suppliers of all types of products who want to implement effective quality systems in their organizations or to improve their existing quality systems. The standards also provide generic requirements against which a customer can evaluate the adequacy of a supplier's quality system. These two roles are complimentary. In the context of programs for quality system registration, as in the European Union, the quality assurance role is more visible, but the business value of both roles is important.

ISO 9001, 9002, and 9003 were developed primarily for two-party contractual situations, to satisfy the customer's quality assurance requirements. The aim is to increase the confidence of customers in the quality systems of their suppliers. This is particularly important when the supplier and the customer are in different countries or when the distance between them is great. This benefit is accomplished by establishing consistent quality practices that cross international borders, providing a common language or set of terms, and minimizing the need for on-site customer visits or audits.

Another aim of the series is to harmonize international trade by supplying a set of standards with worldwide credibility and acceptance. The series has, in fact, become accepted as a *de facto* baseline requirement that is separate from its use within the European Union-regulated industry structure. Manufacturers and service industries report that some standard contract forms now include quality system registration queries.

For some countries, registration to ISO 9001, 9002, or 9003 is a legal requirement to enter the regulated European Union market. Registration might also help a company meet a domestic regulatory mandate.

Legal concerns are also driving registration. Some companies register a quality system, at least in part, for the role ISO 9000 registration may play in product liability defense. Companies that sell regulated products in Western Europe may be subject to increasingly stringent product liability and safety requirements that are moving toward the strict liability concepts prevalent in the United States.

6.3 Structure of the ISO 9000 Standards

The ISO 9000 Series are consensus standards, and by their nature contain quality principles widely accepted in authoritative texts and by expert groups. They provide a yardstick for suppliers of goods and services, including but not limited to FDA regulated products, to measure their capability to supply quality products. There are five standards in the ISO 9000 series:

ISO 9000	The guideline for selection and use of standards ISO 9001, 9002, and 9003.

	Adopted by the European Committee for Standardization (CEN) as a European Standard (EN29000).
ISO 9001	The highest level of quality assurance standard. It contains 20 requirements including design and servicing.
	Adopted by the European Committee for Standardization (CEN) as a European Standard (EN29001).
ISO 9002	The intermediary and most popular level of quality assurance standard. It contains 18 requirements, omitting design and servicing from ISO 9001.
	Adopted by the European Committee for Standardization (CEN) as a European Standard (EN29002).
ISO 9003	The least stringent set of ISO standards. It contains 12 requirements and deals with quality assurance in final inspection and test. This standard is used infrequently in registrations involving manufacturing.
	Adopted by the European Committee for Standardization (CEN) as a European Standard (EN29003).
ISO 9004	An overview of quality assurance system requirements. It includes quality management purposes as well as explaining quality system design.
	Adopted by the European Committee for Standardization (CEN) as a European Standard (EN29004).

Additional ISO 9000 Guidelines have been developed to assist in meeting the five main standards.

ISO 9000-1	Guideline for the selection and use of applicable standards.
ISO 9000-2	Guideline to the application of ISO 9001/9002/9003.
ISO 9000-3	Guideline for the application of ISO 9001 to the development, supply, and maintenance of software.
ISO 9000-4	Guideline on dependability program management.

The usefulness of uniform quality standards on a global scale, except for certain allied military applications, just became widely recognized during the last two decades. Previously, both business and government considered consumer product quality assurance systems as they were applied internally within corporate or other business entities. To develop and document quality systems, using a common approach, facilitates communication between manufacturers or service businesses and their suppliers. There is growing worldwide recognition that total quality management (TQM) provides a superior mechanism for marketplace competitiveness, as opposed to finished product testing or inspection, and this creates the need for parties to communicate reliable quality information. Registration or conformance with the appropriate ISO 9000 standard provides a foundation for quality programs that, to be consistent with TQM, must include both component suppliers and manufacturers.

6.4 The Requirements of the ISO 9000 Standards

The requirements of the ISO 9000 series of standards are classified into 20 different clauses:

- Management Responsibility
- Quality Systems
- Contract Review
- Design Control
- Document and Data Control
- Purchasing

- Control of Customer Supplied Product
- Product Identification and Traceability
- Process Control
- Inspection and Testing
- Test Equipment
- Inspection and Test Status
- Control of Nonconforming Product
- Corrective Action
- Handling, Storage, Packaging, and Delivery
- Quality Records
- Internal Quality Audit
- Training
- Servicing
- Statistical Techniques

Each of these requirements is discussed in detail in Chapter 7.

6.5 The ISO 9000 Registration Process

Regardless of which registrar is selected, the registration process generally consists of the following basic steps:

- Application
- Document review
- Pre-assessment
- Assessment
- Registration
- Surveillance.

6.5.1 Application

To begin the registration process, most registrars require a completed application, sometimes called a contract. The application usually contains the rights and obligations of both the registrar and the client. It should contain such registrar rights as access to facilities, access to necessary information, as well as liability issues. The application should contain such client rights as confidentiality, the right to appeal and complain, and instructions for the use of the registration certificate and associated marks.

Prior to issuing an application, the organization should ensure that the registrar fully understands the extent of the operation to be certified and that the certification is within the registrar's accredited scope. It is also important, especially for large companies with centralized functions that elect to use more than one registrar, to determine each registrar's policy relative to acceptance of registration by another registrar.

6.5.2 Document Review

Once the application is completed with basic information on the company's size, scope of operations, and desired time frame for registration, the registrar typically requests the company to submit documentation of its quality system. This documentation is generally in the format of a Quality Manual. The Quality Manual is a document that describes the overall quality system of the organization as well as how each applicable clause of the standard is met, including the appropriate company document reference numbers.

A sample of the Table of Contents for the typical Quality Manual includes the following topics:

<u>Cross Reference List</u>

A cross reference list of company documentation that addresses each clause of the ISO standard.

<u>Introduction</u>

A description of the company, including site locations, types of products sold, number of employees, organization chart, and the method of establishing the Quality System.

<u>Control</u>

A description of how the Quality Manual is controlled.

<u>Scope of the Quality System</u>

A list of what areas within the company are included in the Quality System.

Distribution

A description of how the Quality Manual is distributed within the company and where the Master Copy resides.

Amendments

A description of how changes are made to the Quality Manual.

ISO Standard Clauses

A description of how each applicable clause of the ISO standard is addressed within the company. For example, a paragraph would be written for each of the following headings under Clause 4.0 Design Control of ISO 9001:

- Design and Development Planning
- Organizational and Technical Interfaces
- Design Input
- Design Output
- Design Verification
- Design Changes.

The paragraphs should indicate that procedures are established and maintained to control the product design activity to ensure that the design requirements are met.

6.5.3 Pre-Assessment

Most registrars recommend that a pre-assessment audit be conducted. Some may require it. A pre-assessment audit is typically a full assessment audit, where the registrar acts as a consultant in determining whether the quality system meets the standard and how particular requirements must be addressed.

A pre-assessment helps identify major system deficiencies, thereby alerting the company to the need for additional preparation prior to the full assessment. Conversely, the organization may have overprepared in some areas, based on its own interpretation of the requirements. An aggressive response to the pre-assessment increases a company's chances of passing the full assessment on the first attempt.

6.5.4 Assessment

In a typical full assessment, two or three auditors spend two to five days at a facility, depending on the size and complexity of the operations to be registered. The auditors will hold an introductory meeting with company management, request escorts to assist them during the audit, hold a closing meeting to communicate any deficiencies that were discovered, and, as appropriate, leave a draft report containing the audit team's findings and recommendation regarding registration. During the audit, the auditors will interview all levels of personnel to determine whether the quality system, as documented in the quality manual and supporting procedures, has been fully implemented within the company.

The assessment audit is discussed in detail in Section 7 of this chapter.

6.5.5 Registration

There are typically three possible results of the assessment audit:

Approval

A company can expect to become registered if it has implemented all the elements of the appropriate ISO standard and only minor deficiencies are detected during the assessment.

Conditional or Provisional Approval

A company can expect to receive conditional or provisional approval if it has addressed all the elements of the appropriate standard and has documented the system, but perhaps has not fully implemented them, or a number of deficiencies detected in a particular area show a negative, systemic trend. Conditional approval requires the company to respond to any deficiencies noted during a time frame defined by the registrar. The registrar, upon evaluating the company's corrective action, may elect to perform an on-site reevaluation or accept the corrective action in writing and review the implementation in conjunction with subsequent surveillance visits.

Disapproval

Disapproval occurs when a company's system is either very well documented but has not been implemented, or when entire elements of the standard have not been addressed at all. This is known as a major deficiency. One major deficiency will cause a disapproval. This situation will require a comprehensive reevaluation by the registrar prior to issuing an approval.

Once a company is registered, it receives a certificate and is listed in a register or directory published by the registrar or another organization. The company should also expect to receive rules for use of the certificate and associated quality marks at this time.

6.5.6 Surveillance

The duration and/or validity of a company's registration may vary. Some registrars offer registrations that are valid indefinitely, pending continued successful surveillance audits. Other registrars offer registrations valid for a specific period of time, such as three or four years.

Most registrars conduct surveillance audits every six months or every twelve months. These surveillance audits usually consist of only a portion of a standard's requirements. Those whose registrations expire conduct either a complete reassessment at the end of the registration period, or an assessment that is somewhere between a surveillance visit and a complete re-audit. It is important for the company to clearly understand the registrar's policy in this area.

During the interval between surveillance visits, the company should continually ensure that its demonstrated quality systems remain in place, so that the surveillance audit will merely confirm that fact. The company should also strive for continual improvement.

6.6 Choosing a Registrar

A key issue for companies selecting registrars is whether a registrar is accredited. Accreditation is the initial evaluation and periodic monitoring of a registrar. It is performed by an accreditation body. Registrars can be accredited by more than one accreditation body. In this case, the company has the opportunity to choose the registration scheme under which it wishes to participate.

When choosing a registrar, several important characteristics need to be considered:

- the marketplace of the company and customer requirements
- conflict of interest if a registrar offers and performs consulting and assessment or registration services
- the total cost of the registration process
- the financial stability of the registrar
- background checks and policies of the registrar
- auditor qualifications
- frequency of recertification audits
- the company's schedule.

6.7 The Certification Audit

The typical ISO 9000 audit consists of the following steps:

- the third party receives and reviews the organization's Quality Manual
- the lead auditor establishes the agenda for the audit and shares it with the organization
- the auditors arrive on site and meet first with the executive staff
- auditing of the individual areas begins with the assistance of company supplied escorts
- summary meetings are held at the end of each day, where auditors review the days findings with each other and then with the company's ISO team
- at the conclusion of the audit, a concluding meeting with

the executive staff is held where each discrepancy is discussed along with the time table for the companies response to each

- the lead auditor sets a tentative schedule for the recertification audit
- the recommendation of the audit team for approval or disapproval is discussed.

The auditors need to review the Quality Manual to familiarize themselves with the company, its organization and how it meets each of the requirements of the applicable standard.

The agenda for the audit is a breakdown of which areas are to be covered and the time frame involved.

The opening meeting, held with the executive staff, is to introduce the members of the audit team to the executive staff and vice versa, to discuss the purpose of the audit, to review the agenda, and to discuss the purpose of the closing meeting.

One or two employees will accompany each auditor. The primary accompanier can intercede where necessary, more fully explain an answer, and/or suggest changing interviewees. The secondary accompanier can take notes. The secondary accompanier usually makes no comments during the audit. The goals for all escorts are to help present the quality system in its best possible light, protect the company's interest, and obtain certification.

During the initial assessment audit, all clauses from the appropriate standard are audited. Based on the agenda, an auditor may spend 1/2 to 1 hour on a particular topic. If a problem is found, the auditor may spend more time. During surveillance audits, only a portion of the total number of clauses, usually 50% are audited.

During the audit, the auditors may speak with anyone working in a particular area. Part-time or contract employees are considered the same as full time employees and they are expected to answer the same questions. Each employee should know the company's quality policy statement and the name of the ISO management representative. Some companies have printed both items on a business card-sized paper and enclosed it in plastic for easy reference. Others have placed the two items on the company's computer network so that they appear when the computer first begins to operate.

Three of the most popular questions to ask are:

- What do you do?
- Where is the procedure that tells you how to do what you do?
- Where is the proof that you follow the procedure?

Each employee should be honest and direct in answering the auditor's questions. They should answer only the question that is asked and not volunteer information which has not been asked. Auditors find trails to problem areas by information that has been volunteered or by hearing talk while walking through a particular area. Some of the most frequently asked questions by auditors are:

- How does you job affect quality?
- Do you work to procedures?
- Where are the procedures?
- Show me the procedure for this job function.
- How do you know this is the latest/most current revision of the procedure?
- Is your equipment calibrated?
- What do you do when things go wrong?
- How do you handle nonconforming product?
- What kind of training have you had?
- What king of ISO training have you had?
- What is the quality policy that governs your work?

At the end of each day, the auditors will meet by themselves and discuss the findings for the day. They may take the time to write up the non-conformance report at that time.

Auditors will usually meet with the escorts and other members of the ISO team following their meeting to review the findings of the day. Any non-conformances should not be a surprise to the escorts, as the auditor should have indicated they have found a discrepancy at the time it is noted. The company may also, at this time, report any corrective actions that have been completed regarding nonconformances found earlier. The auditors will still report the nonconformance, but will indicate it has been corrected.

At the conclusion of the audit, the lead auditor will conduct a closing meeting to discuss the findings of the audit with the executive staff and other employees of the company. Each nonconformance will be discussed and the company representative asked to sign the report. The company may at this time express any disagreements with the findings. Sometimes a company is successful in having a nonconformance reclassified. The lead auditor will also indicate a time frame for submitting corrective action. Based on the severity and number of nonconformances, corrective action may be sent to the auditor or a re-audit may be necessary. The lead auditor may also indicate the recommendation for certification or noncertification at this time. The lead auditor thanks the company representatives for their assistance in the audit and the audit team leaves.

To successfully survive an assessment audit, there are several general rules which should be observed. In addition to preparing well in advance of the actual audit and learning from gap assessment and pre-assessment audits, these rules are a common sense approach to the process:

- Say what you do
- Do what you say
- Prove it
- Keep documents simple
- Be honest with the auditor
- Ensure obsolete documents are removed
- Identify legitimate copies of Standard Operating Procedures by some means, such as colored paper
- Contract or temporary personnel are considered the same as full time employees - they must know the same information:
    - The company's quality policy.
    - The management representative.
    - How does their job affect quality?

Despite the best efforts of any company, the auditors will usually find some nonconformances. These are usually minor nonconformances and do not threaten the certification to be achieved. Some of the more common nonconformances found in ISO 9001 audits include:

- Lack of knowledge of individual responsibilities
- Interfaces
- Lack of master list or equivalent document control procedure to identify current revision
- Lack of ownership of quality records
- No written instructions or information
- Failure to follow instructions
- Unauthorized changes

- Lack of removal of obsolete documents
- Ineffective corrective action
- Lack of support for corrective action
- Uncalibrated equipment
- Rework or repair not done
- No documented procedures in measurement and inspection
- No calibration labeling
- Calibration intervals not controlled
- Lack of system in measurement and inspection
- Lack of adequate training records
- Lack of connection between procedures and instructions.

Knowing these and preparing for them in advance will increase the possibility of achieving certification.

6.8 ISO 9000 Costs

The costs of certifying to one of the ISO 9000 series of standards will vary depending on the size of the organization and the Notified Body that is chosen. The following costs for certification are based on an average of many types of manufacturers:

- The average time to prepare for the assessment audit was 18 months
- The average cost for a Notified Body was $21,000
- The average total cost for the certification process, including internal costs and auditing fees, was $245,200
- The average time to recoup the cost of registration was 40 months.

As an example of an individual industry, average costs for a computer company for registration were:

Internal costs	$164,200
External costs	43,200
Notified Body	23,200
Total	$230, 600

In comparison, the costs for a chemical company averaged:

Internal costs	$301,500
External costs	50,500
Notified Body	23,300
Total	$374,900

6.9 ISO 9000 and the FDA

The Center for Devices and Radiological Health (CDRH) has extensive experience working with standards organizations, both nationally and internationally. This is due in part to their application of the performance standards requirements of the Radiation Control for Health and Safety Act of 1968 and in part to the standards provisions of the Medical Device Amendments of 1976. The Safe Medical Devices Act of 1990 (SMDA) obligated CDRH to establish an Office of International Regulations and authorized the Secretary to enter into agreements with foreign countries to facilitate international trade in medical devices and to encourage the mutual recognition of good manufacturing practice regulations, other regulations, and testing protocols deemed appropriate.

The Office of Standards and Regulations in CDRH has reported, annually for the fast few years, their standards development activities. CDRH has assigned personnel to national and international technical and management committees and involved scientists from other agency components when necessary. CDRH reported at the end of October, 1992 that over 177 staff members were working intermittently on 371 different standards with 31 different organizations. Ninety-one of these were under the auspices of seven international organizations. In the past, the development of international standards for medical devices was focused on vertical standards. However, current philosophy is that horizontal standards, such as the ISO 9000 series, are more flexible and thus consensus can be achieved more readily.

The recent Quality System Regulations are modeled after the ISO 9000 series. Each clause in the ISO document is addressed in the Quality System Regulation.

References

Fries, Richard C., *Reliable Design of Medical Devices.* New York: Marcel Dekker, Inc., 1997.

Lynch, Mark A. and William L. Schwemer, "ISO 9000 Policy Implementation for FDA - Taking the Pulse of Increasing Global Use of the ISO Series of Uniform Quality Standards by FDA Regulated Industries," *Regulatory Affairs*. Spring, 1993.

Peach, Robert W., *The ISO 9000 Handbook. 2nd Edition.* Fairfax, Virginia: CEEM Information Services, 1995.

Todorov, Branimir, *ISO 9000 Required: Your Worldwide Passport to Customer Confidence.* Portland, Oregon: Productivity Press, 1996.

Zaloom, Victor, *ISO 9000 Standards Implementation.* Beaumont, Texas: Industrial Engineering Systems, 1995.

Chapter 7

ISO 9000 Requirements

The ISO 9000 series of standards deal with quality system requirements that can be used for external quality assurance purposes. The series consist of three documents:

ISO 9001	For use when conformance to specified requirements is to be ensured during design, development, production, installation, and servicing
ISO 9002	For use when conformance to specified requirements is to be ensured during production, installation, and servicing
ISO 9003	For use when conformance to specified requirements is to be ensured at final inspection and test.

This chapter covers all requirements as listed in ISO 9001. For those readers interested in ISO 9002 or 9003, they should review only the appropriate clauses.

7.1 Management Responsibility

7.1.1 Requirements

This clause has the following requirements:

- Senior management must define and document its quality policies and objectives and commit to them
- Management must ensure the policies and objectives are communicated effectively throughout the organization
- Management must define the responsibility, authority, and interrelationships of all personnel affecting the quality of products or services
- Adequate resources and trained personnel must be available to carry out any verification work
- Regular management reviews of the system must be conducted to ensure the system is functioning effectively
- A management representative must be identified and given sufficient authority to manage the system on a day-to-day basis.

7.1.2 Compliance

7.1.2.1 Quality Policy

The Quality Policy is the overall intentions and direction of an organization with regard to quality as formally expressed by top management.

The quality policy must be:

- easy to understand
- relevant to the organization
- ambitious, yet achievable.

To fulfill the requirement, management must define the quality policy, quality objectives, and quality commitment of the organization. Once defined, the policy, objectives and commitment must be documented. Management must then ensure everyone in the organization understands, implements, and maintains the quality policy. This can be accomplished by posting a copy of the quality policy in frequently used places within the organization, printing cards with the quality policy that employees can carry with them, or providing training programs where the quality policy is emphasized.

7.1.2.2 Organization

The organization is required to define the responsibility, authority and the interrelation of all personnel affecting the quality of product and service to customers. Individuals in the organization should:

- be aware of the scope, responsibility and authority of their functions
- be aware of the impact on product and service quality
- have adequate authority to carry out their responsibilities
- understand clearly their defined authority
- accept responsibility for achieving quality objectives.

7.1.2.3 Resources

Once policies and objectives are defined, adequate resources and trained personnel must be available to fulfill the commitment to achieve the policies and objectives. Management must provide sufficient resources to develop and maintain the quality management system. These people must be properly trained, either through education, experience, and/or on-site training. Records of the training must be kept on file.

7.1.2.4 Management Review

Management must conduct regular management reviews of the qualiy management system to make sure it remains suitable and effective. These reviews must be held on a regular, defined basis and all reviews documented. Where action items are developed, personnel and time frames for completion should be identified.

The scope of management reviews should normally discuss, at a minimum, the following topics:

- organizational structure
- implementation of the quality system
- the achieved quality of the product or service
- information based on customer feedback, internal audits, process and product performance.

7.1.2.5 Management Representative

A management representative must be appointed who has authority to implement and maintain the quality system. If the management representative has other functions, there should be no conflict of interest with those functions. The management representative should be trained in the details of ISO 9000 and be prepared to coordinate all activities necessary to develop and maintain the quality management system.

7.2 Quality Systems

7.2.1 Requirements

This clause has the following requirements:

- The quality management system must be documented
- A Quality Manual and Quality Plans need to be created
- Quality system procedures and instructions must be produced
- Quality system procedures and instructions must be effectively implemented.

7.2.2 Compliance

7.2.2.1 Documented System

The quality management system must be documented. Documentation should include preparatory work to develop the quality management system, the details of how the quality management system will be implemented, and how the quality management system will be maintained. The documentation of the quality management system is normally done in the form of the Quality Manual and Quality Plans.

7.2.2.2 Quality Manual and Quality Plans

The Quality Manual is a document that describes the organization's overall quality system and how each applicable clause of the standard is met, including appropriate company document reference numbers. The typical Quality Manual would contain the following sections:

Cross Reference List	a cross reference list of company documentation that addresses each clause of the ISO 9000 standard.
Introduction	a description of the company, including site locations, types of products sold, number of employees, organization chart, and the method of establishing and maintaining the quality management system.
Control	a description of how the Quality Manual is controlled.
Scope	a list of what areas within the organization will be included in the quality management system.
Distribution	a description of how the Quality Manual is distributed within the organization and the location of the master copy of the Quality Manual.
Amendments	a description of how changes are made to the Quality Manual.
ISO Clauses	a description of how each applicable clause of the ISO 9000 standard is addressed within the organization. The description should indicate that procedures are established and maintained to ensure the requirements of the particular clause are met.

Quality plans should be developed as appropriate to address individual requirements. Quality plans may be in the form of a reference to the appropriate documented procedures that form an integral part of the quality management system.

7.2.2.3 Documented Control/Maintenance

Controlled procedures must be established that address, at a minimum, each clause of the ISO 9000 standard. Procedures are an overall description of a particular activity.

Controlled work instructions must be established that list the details involved in performing the activity listed in a procedure.

7.2.2.4 Effective Implementation

Effective implementation of procedures and work instructions must be ensured and documented. Once the procedures and work instructions have been written, the requirements of the documentation should be periodically audited and the results discussed and acted upon during the management review.

7.3 Contract Review

7.3.1 Requirements

This clause has the following requirements:

- Procedures for contract review must be established and maintained
- Procedures for coordination of contract review activities must be established and maintained
- Each contract must adequately define and document the requirements
- Each contract must resolve any requirements differing from those in the tender
- The manufacturer must ensure that the supplier has the capability to meet contractual requirements
- Records of contract review must be maintained.

7.3.2 Compliance

7.3.2.1 Contract Review Procedures

Procedures for review of each contract must be established and a process established for maintaining them. Contract review procedures should include:

- a definition of the requirements
- the establishment of a method for resolving differences
- the establishment of a method for ensuring the supplier has the capability to meet contract requirements.

Records of review must be documented and maintained.

7.3.2.2 Procedures for Coordination of Contract Review Activities

Procedures for establishing and maintaining a contract review process must be developed and maintained. The basic elements of the contract review process include:

- ensuring the scope of the contract is clearly defined
- adequately documenting thc requirements
- identifying and resolving any variations
- ensuring the capability to fulfill the contract exists
- ensuring the technical skills exist in-house or can be acquired
- verify the work can be done for the price
- ensure the work can be delivered according to requirements
- ensuring any amendments to the contract are effectively handled.

7.3.2.3 Requirements

Requirements of the contract review must be adequately defined and documented. The requirements must be understood by both the manufacturer and the supplier. Where no written statement of requirement is available for a verbal order, the supplier must ensure the order requirements are agreed before the acceptance.

Any differences between contract or accepted order requirements and those in the tender must be resolved between the manufacturer and the supplier. Resolution of differences must be documented.

7.3.2.4 Supplier Selection

Suppliers of components, products, or services must be selected on the basis of their ability to meet the requirements of the defined component, product, or service. Most selections are based on a review of the supplier's product as well as an audit of the supplier, at his location. Such supplier audits include reviews of:

- the supplier's quality management system
- documentation controls
- process capability
- component, product, or service reliability
- the stability of the business
- the supplier's financial situation.

All audits of suppliers should be documented and maintained.

7.4 Design Control

7.4.1 Requirements

Design control has the following requirements:

- Management must establish and maintain procedures to control and verify the design of the product
- Plans must be developed that identify the responsibility for each design and development activity
- Design and verification activities must be planned and assigned to qualified personnel equipped with adequate resources
- Organizational and technical interfaces between different groups must be identified and the necessary information documented, transmitted, and regularly reviewed
- Design input requirements must be identified, documented, and their selection reviewed

- Design output must be documented and expressed in terms of requirements, calculations, and analyses
- Formal documented reviews of the design results shall be planned and conducted at appropriate stages of the design
- Management must plan, establish, document and assign to competent personnel functions for verifying the design
- Procedures for the identification, documentation, and appropriate review and approval must be established for all changes and modifications
- A procedure for developing and maintaining a list of active design projects and their status must be established and maintained.

7.4.2 Compliance

7.4.2.1 Design Procedures

Procedures covering the control and validation of the product design must be established and maintained. The procedures should list the major phases of the product development process. A typical product development process includes:

• feasibility	defining the product to be developed
• design	designing the product from the requirements
• validation	verifying and validating that the new product meets the requirements
• manufacturing	building the product from the design
• field operation	monitoring the operation of the product in the field.

7.4.2.2 Design Plans

Plans for each design and development activity must be established and maintained. Typical plans include:

- description of the activity
- schedule for completion

- list of responsible personnel
- details on the implementation of the plan.

Design plans should be updated as the design evolves.

7.4.2.3 Qualified Personnel

Design, verification, and validation activities must be assigned to personnel who are qualified to perform the required activities. Qualification can be based upon education, experience, and/or on-the-job training. Qualifications of personnel must be documented and maintained.

7.4.2.4 Organizational Interfaces

Interfaces between various parts of the organization involved in the design and development of a product must be documented. The interface documents must be transmitted, maintained by all groups, and regularly reviewed to ensure they are current. Interface documents should include the names of each group involved in the product design and development, and the responsibilities associated with each of them.

7.4.2.5 Design Inputs

Design input requirements, including such items as applicable statutory and regulatory requirements, must be identified, documented, reviewed, and maintained. Incomplete, ambiguous, or conflicting requirements must be resolved with those responsible for imposing the requirements.

Design inputs will take into consideration the results of any contract review activities.

7.4.2.6 Design Outputs

Design outputs must be documented and expressed in terms that can be verified against design input requirements and validated. Design outputs must:

- meet the design input requirements
- contain or make reference to acceptance criteria
- identify those characteristics of the design that are crucial

to the safe and effective functioning of the product. These may include storage, operating, handling, maintenance and disposal requirements.

Design outputs must be reviewed and maintained.

7.4.2.7 Design Reviews

Formal design reviews are generally held according to the project plan and are convened to support major project milestones. Design reviews are held to highlight critical aspects of the design and focus attention on possible shortfalls. The primary purpose of the design review is to make a choice among alternative design approaches. The output of the review should include an understanding of the weak areas in the design and the areas of the design in need of special attention.

The typical design review should include a discussion of:

- redundancy versus derating
- redesign of weak areas versus high reliability parts
- Failure Mode and Effects Analysis (FMEA) activity
- potential product misuse
- overstressed parts.

Design reviews should follow a structured order and be well documented, including topics discussed, decisions reached, resulting action items, personnel responsible for the action items, and a schedule for addressing the action items.

Design review personnel should not have taken part in the actual design activity, as this gives a fresh and unbiased look at the design. Reviewers should understand they have a serious responsibility to comment on the potential outcome of the project and understand project objectives and product requirements. Participants must include representatives of all functions concerned with the design stage being reviewed, as well as other specialist personnel, as required.

7.4.2.8 Verification and Validation

At appropriate stages of the design, design verification must be performed to ensure that the particular design stage meets the design-stage input requirements. Verification activity must be documented, including verification protocol, test unit setup, details of the activity, results, an indication of acceptance or failure, personnel performing the activity, and the date the activity was performed.

Design validation must be performed to ensure that the product conforms to the defined requirements. The validation activity must be documented including validation protocol, requirements being tested, test unit setup, details of the activity, results, an indication of acceptance or failure, personnel performing the activity, and the date the activity was performed.

Verification, and validation activities must be assigned to personnel who are qualified to perform the required activities. Qualification can be based upon education, experience, and/or on-the job training. Qualifications of personnel must be documented and maintained.

7.4.2.9 Design Changes

Procedures must be established and maintained that detail the design change process. The documentation must address how design changes are identified, documented, reviewed and approved prior to implementation. The list of those individuals authorized to review and approve changes should be kept on file.

7.4.2.10 List of Current Design Activities

A procedure for developing and maintaining a list of current design activities and their status with respect to the defined product development process must be established and maintained. The list must be available to be reviewed by the ISO auditor.

7.5 Document and Data Control

7.5.1 Requirements

This clause has the following requirements:

- Procedures must be established and maintained to control all documents and data
- Documents and data must be reviewed and approved for adequacy by authorized personnel prior to issue

- A master list or equivalent document-control procedure identifying the current revision status of documents must be established and readily available
- Changes to documents and data must be reviewed and approved by the same functions/organizations that performed the original review and approval, unless specifically designated otherwise.

7.5.2 Compliance

7.5.2.1 Document and Data Procedures

Procedures must be established and maintained that describe the control of all documents and data. Documents and data can be in the form of any type of media, including hard copy or electronic media. Control must ensure:

- the pertinent issues of appropriate documents are available at all locations where operations essential to the effective functioning of the quality management system are performed
- invalid and/or other obsolete documents are promptly removed from all points of issue or use, or otherwise ensured against unintended use
- any obsolete documents retained for legal and/or knowledge preservation purposes are suitably identified.

Internal written procedures should contain how documentation for these functions should be controlled, who is responsible for document control, what is to be controlled, and where and when is it to be controlled.

Documents and data must be reviewed and approved for adequacy by authorized personnel prior to issue.

7.5.2.2 Master List

A master list or equivalent document-control procedure identifying the current revision status of documents must be established and be readily available to preclude the use of invalid and/or obsolete documents.

7.5.2.3 Document and Data Changes

Changes to documents and data shall be reviewed and approved by the same functions that performed the original review and approval, unless specifically designated otherwise. The change process includes:

- review and approval
- access to background information
- the nature of the change identified
- review of the master list or equivalent
- review of the number of changes that have occurred to the document or data.

7.6 Purchasing

7.6.1 Requirements

Purchasing has the following requirements:

- Procedures must be established and maintained to ensure that purchased product conforms to specified requirements
- Suppliers must be evaluated on the basis of their ability to meet contract requirements
- Purchasing documents shall contain data clearly describing the product ordered
- Purchasing documents must be reviewed and approved for adequacy of the specified requirements
- Verification arrangements and the method of product release must be specified
- Where verified in the contract, the customer must be afforded the right to verify that the product conforms to specified requirements.

7.6.2 Compliance

Conformance to requirements is a supplier responsibility.

7.6.2.1 Procedures

Procedures must be established and maintained to ensure that purchased product conforms to specified requirements.

7.6.2.2 Vendor Evaluation

Vendors must be evaluated and selected on the basis of their ability to meet contract requirements including the quality system and any specific quality assurance requirements. Vendor evaluation should address:

- their ability to meet requirements
- comparison to records of acceptable vendors.

Vendor evaluations must address

- previous performance in supplying similar products
- satisfactory assessment of an appropriate quality system standard by a competent body
- assessment of the vendor by the manufacturer to an appropriate quality system standard
- product compliance with specified requirements
- total cost for the vendor
- delivery arrangements
- periodic review of the performance of the vendor.

The manufacturer must define the type and extent of control it exercises over its vendors. This is dependent upon the type of product, the impact of vended product on the quality of the final product, and, where applicable, on the quality audit reports and/or quality records of the previously demonstrated capability and performance of vendors. Control depends on:

- the type of product
- records of performance.

The manufacturer must also establish and maintain quality records of acceptable vendors.

7.6.2.3 Purchasing Documents

Purchasing documents must contain data clearly describing the product ordered, including:

- the type, class, grade, or other precise identification
- the title or other positive identification, and applicable issues of :
  - specifications
  - drawings
  - process requirements
  - inspection instructions
  - other relevant technical data
- the title, number, and issue of the quality-system standard to be applied.

Purchasing documents must be reviewed and approved for adequacy of the specified requirements.

7.6.2.4 Verification Arrangements

Where the vendor proposes to verify purchased product at the vendor's premises, the manufacturer shall specify verification arrangements and the method of product release in the purchasing documents.

Where specified in the contract, the vendor's customer or the customer's representative must be afforded the right to verify at the vendor's premises that the contracted product conforms to specified requirements. Such verification shall not be used by the manufacturer as evidence of effective control of quality by the subcontractor.

Verification by the manufacturer shall not absolve the vendor of the responsibility to provide acceptable product, nor shall it preclude subsequent rejection by the manufacturer.

7.7 Control of Customer-Supplied Product

7.7.1 Requirements

This clause has the following requirements:

- Procedures must be established and maintained for the control of verification, storage, and maintenance of customer-supplied product.

7.7.2 Compliance

Customer-supplied product is any product owned by the customer and furnished to the supplier for use in meeting the requirements of the contract. The supplier must establish and maintain procedures for maintaining the quality of product supplied by the purchaser. Records must be kept and reports made of any such product that is lost, damaged, or unsuitable for use.

7.8 Product Identification and Traceability

7.8.1 Requirements

This clause has the following requirements:

- Where appropriate, procedures must be established and maintained for identifying the product from suitable means from receipt and during all stages of production, delivery, and installation
- When traceability is a specified requirement, procedures must be established and maintained for unique identification of individual product or batches.

7.8.2 Compliance

Where appropriate, the supplier shall establish procedures for identifying the product during all stages of production, delivery, and installation. Where traceability is a specific requirement, individual production batches shall have unique identification. This identification shall be recorded.

7.9 Process Control

7.9.1 Requirements

Process control has the following requirements:

- Production, installation, and servicing processes must be identified and planned
- Management must ensure these processes are carried out under controlled conditions
- Where the results of processes cannot be fully verified by subsequent inspection and testing of the product, the process must be carried out by qualified operators and/or shall require continuous monitoring and control of process parameters
- Records must be maintained for qualified processes, equipment, and personnel, as appropriate.

7.9.2 Compliance

7.9.2.1 Identification and Planning

The manufacturer must identify and plan the production, installation, and servicing processes which directly affect quality. The supplier is required to identify and plan the processing steps needed to produce the product, ensure that the processes are carried out under controlled conditions, provide documented instructions for work that affects quality, monitor and approve necessary processes, observe and stipulate relevant criteria for workmanship, and where practical, maintain equipment to ensure continuing process capability.

Companies should also conduct process capability studies to determine the potential effectiveness of a process, develop work instructions that describe the criteria for determining satisfactory work, verify the quality status of a product, process, software, material, or environment, verify the capability of production processes in accordance with specifications, control and verify auxiliary materials and utilities, such as water, compressed air, electric power, and chemicals used for processing where they are important to quality characteristics.

7.9.2.2 Controlled Conditions

The manufacturer must ensure the identified processes are carried out under controlled conditions. Controlled conditions include:

- documented procedures defining the manner of production, installation, and servicing, where the absence of such procedures could adversely affect quality
- use of suitable production, installation, and servicing equipment, and a suitable working environment
- compliance with reference standards/codes, quality plans, and/or documented procedures
- monitoring and control of suitable process parameters and product characteristics
- the approval of processes and equipment, as appropriate
- criteria for workmanship, which must be stipulated in the clearest practical manner
- suitable maintenance of equipment to ensure continuing process capability.

7.9.2.3 Lack of Full Verification

Where the results of processes cannot be fully verified by subsequent inspection and testing of the product, Where, for example, processing efficiencies may become apparent only after the product is in use, the processes must be carried out by qualified operators and/or must require continuous monitoring and control of process parameters to ensure that the specified requirements are met. The requirements for any qualification or process operations, including personnel and associated equipment, must be specified.

7.9.2.4 Records

Records must be maintained for qualified processes, equipment, and personnel, as appropriate.

7.9.2.5 Special Processes

Special processes are those whose results cannot be fully verified by subsequent inspection and testing of the product and where processing deficiencies may become apparent only after the product is in use. Special processes may require comprehensive measurement assurance and equipment calibration, statistical process control, and special training.

7.10 Inspection and Testing

7.10.1 Requirements

This clause has the following requirements:

- Procedures must be established and maintained for inspection and testing activities
- The required inspection, testing, and records must be detailed in the quality plan or documented procedures
- Incoming product must not be used or processed until it has been inspected or otherwise verified as conforming to specified requirements
- In determining the amount of and nature of receiving inspection, consideration must be given to the amount of control exercised by the supplier
- Where incoming product is released for urgent production purposed prior to verification, it must be positively identified and recorded
- Product must be inspected and tested as required by the quality plan and/or documented procedures
- Product must be held until the required inspection and tests have been completed
- All final inspection and testing must be carried out in accordance with the quality plan and/or documented procedures
- No product shall be dispatched until all activities specified in the quality plan and/or documented procedures have been satisfactorily completed and the associated data and documentation authorized.

7.10.2 Compliance

7.10.2.1 Procedures

The supplier must establish and maintain documented procedures for inspection and testing activities in order to verify that the specified requirements for the product are met. The required inspection and testing, and the records established, must be detailed in the quality plan or documented procedures.

7.10.2.2 Records

Records must be established and maintained which provide evidence that the product has been inspected and/or tested. These records must show clearly whether the product has passed or failed the inspections and/or tests according to defined acceptance criteria. Where the product fails to pass, the procedures for control of nonconforming product must apply. Records must also identify the inspection authority responsible for the release of product.

7.10.2.3 Receiving Inspection and Testing

The manufacturer must ensure that incoming products are not used or processed until they have been inspected or otherwise verified as conforming to specified requirements. Verification of the specified requirements must be in accordance with the quality plan and the documented procedures. In determining the amount and nature of receiving inspection and testing, consideration must be given to the amount of control exercised at the vendor's premises and the recorded evidence of conformance provided.

7.10.2.4 In-Process Inspection and Testing

The manufacturer must inspect and test the product as required by the quality plan and/or documented procedures. The manufacturer must also hold product until the required inspection and tests have been completed or necessary reports have been received and verified. The exception to this requirement is when product is released under positive-recall procedures.

7.10.2.5 Final Inspection and Testing

The manufacturer must carry out all final inspection and testing in accordance with the quality plan and/or documented procedures to complete the evidence of conformance of the finished product to the specified requirements. The quality plan or documented procedures must ensure that all specified inspection and tests, including those specified either on receipt of product or in-process, have been carried out and that the results meet specified requirements.

No product must be dispatched until all the activities specified in the quality plan or documented procedures have been satisfactorily completed and the associated data and documentation are available and authorized.

7.10.2.6 Urgent Production

Where incoming product is released for urgent production purposes prior to verification, it shall be positively identified and recorded in order to permit immediate recall and replacement in the event of nonconformity to specified requirements. The supplier's procedures should include 1) defining responsibilities and authority of people who may allow incoming product to be used without prior demonstration of conformance to specified requirements and 2) explaining how such product will be positively identified and controlled in the event that subsequent inspection finds nonconformities.

7.11 Control of Inspection, Measuring, and Test Equipment

7.11.1 Requirements

This clause has the following requirements:

- Procedures must be established and maintained to control, calibrate, and maintain inspection, measuring, and test equipment, including test software
- Inspection, measuring, and test equipment must be used in a manner that ensures the measurement uncertainty is known and is consistent with the required measurement capability
- Software or comparative references must be checked to ensure they are capable of verifying the acceptability of product, prior to release for use during the production, installation, or servicing of the product
- Software or comparative references must be checked at prescribed intervals
- When the availability of technical data pertaining to the measurement equipment is a specified requirement, such data must be made available when required by the customer or the customer's representative
- Management must determine the measurements to be made and the accuracy required

- Management must identify all inspection, measuring, and test equipment that can affect product quality and calibrate and adjust them at prescribed intervals
- Management must define the process employed for the calibration of inspection, measuring, and test equipment
- Management must identify inspection, measuring, and test equipment with a suitable indicator
- Calibration records must be maintained for inspection, measuring, and test equipment
- Management must assess and document the validity of previous inspections and test results when inspection, measuring, and test equipment is found to be out of calibration
- The handling, preservation and storage of inspection, measuring, and test equipment must be such that the accuracy and fitness for use are maintained
- Management must safeguard inspection, measuring, and test facilities from adjustments that would invalidate the calibration setting.

7.11.2 Compliance

7.11.2.1 Procedures

Documented procedures must be established and maintained to control, calibrate, and maintain inspection, measuring, and test equipment, including test software, used by the manufacturer to demonstrate the conformance of product to the specified requirements. Inspection, measuring, and test equipment must be used in a manner that ensures that the measurement uncertainty is known and is consistent with the required measurement capability.

Where the availability of technical data pertaining to the measurement equipment is a specified requirement, the data must be made available, when required by the customer's representative for verification that the measuring equipment is functionally adequate.

The manufacture must:

- determine the measurements to be made and the accuracy required
- select the appropriate inspection, measuring, and test

equipment that is capable of the necessary accuracy and precision

- identify all inspection, measuring, and test equipment that can affect product quality, and calibrate and adjust them at prescribed intervals, or prior to use, against certified equipment having a known valid relationship to internationally or nationally recognized standards
- document the basis used for calibration where no recognized standards exist
- define the process employed for the calibration of equipment including:
  - details of equipment type
  - unique identification
  - location
  - frequency of checks
  - check method
  - acceptance criteria
  - the action to be taken when results are not satisfactory
- identify equipment with a suitable indicator or approved identification record to show the calibration status
- maintain calibration records for inspection, measuring, and test equipment
- assess and document the validity of previous inspection and test results when equipment is found to be out of calibration
- ensure that the environmental conditions are suitable for the calibrations, inspections, measurements, and tests being carried out
- ensure that the handling, preservation, and storage of inspection, measuring, and test equipment is such that the accuracy and fitness for use are maintained
- safeguard inspection, measuring, and test facilities, including both test hardware and test software, from adjustments which would invalidate the calibration setting.

7.11.2.2 Test Software and Hardware

Where test software or comparative references such as test hardware are used as suitable forms of inspection, they must be checked to prove that they are capable of verifying the acceptability of product prior to release for use during production, installation, or servicing, and must be rechecked at prescribed intervals.

7.12 Inspection and Test Status

7.12.1 Requirements

This clause has the following requirements:

- The inspection and test status of product shall be identified by suitable means, which indicate the conformance or nonconformance of product with regard to inspection and tests performed
- The identification of inspection and test status must be maintained as defined in the quality plan and/or documented procedures

7.12.2 Compliance

7.12.2.1 Identification

The inspection and test status of a product must be identified by a suitable means, which indicate the conformance or nonconformance of product with regard to inspection and tests performed. The identification of inspection and test status must be maintained as defined in the quality plan and/or documented procedures, throughout production, installation, and servicing of the product to ensure that only product that has passed the required inspections and tests is dispatched, used, or installed.

Status should indicate whether the product has:

- not been inspected
- been inspected and accepted
- been inspected and on hold awaiting decision
- been inspected and rejected.

Identification should indicate:

- verified versus unverified material
- acceptance at the point of verification
- traceability to the unit responsible for the operation.

7.13 Control of Nonconforming Product

7.13.1 Requirements

This clause has the following requirements:

- Procedures must be established and maintained to ensure product that does not conform to specified requirements is prevented from unintended use or installation
- The control must provide for identification, documentation, evaluation, segregation, disposition, and notification to appropriate functions
- The responsibility for review and authority for the disposition of nonconforming product must be defined
- Nonconforming product must be reviewed in accordance with documented procedures
- When required by the contract, the proposed use or repair of product which does not conform to specified requirements must be reported for concession
- Repaired and/or reworked product must be reinspected in accordance with the quality plan and/or documented prodcedures.

7.13.2 Compliance

7.13.2.1 Procedures

Documented procedures must be established and maintained to ensure that product that does not conform to specified requirements is prevented from unintended use or installation. The manufacturer must ensure such nonconforming product is identified, documented, evaluated, segregated, and disposed of. Notification of the nonconformity must be made to the functions concerned.

Procedures for controlling non-conforming product should include:

- determining which product units are involved in the non-conformity
- identifying the nonconforming product units
- documenting the nonconformity
- evaluating the nonconformity

- considering alternatives for disposing of the non-conforming product units
- physically controlling the movement, storage, and processing of the nonconforming product units
- notifying all functions that may be affected by the non-conformity.

7.13.2.2 Review and Disposition of Nonconforming Product

The responsibility for review and authority for the disposition of nonconforming product must be defined. Nonconforming product must be reviewed in accordance with documented procedures. Nonconforming product may be:

- reworked to meet the specified requirements, per documented procedures
- accepted with or without repair by concession
- re-graded for alternative applications
- rejected or scrapped.

Repaired and/or reworked product must be reinspected in accordance with the quality plan and/or documented procedures.

7.14 Corrective and Preventive Action

7.14.1 Requirements

This clause has the following requirements:

- Procedures must be established and maintained for implementing corrective and preventive action
- Any corrective or preventive action taken to eliminate the causes of actual or potential nonconformities must be to a degree appropriate to the magnitude of problems and commensurate with the risks encountered.

7.14.2 Compliance

7.14.2.1 Procedures

Documented procedures must be established and maintained for implementing corrective and preventive action. Any corrective action taken to eliminate the causes of actual or potential nonconformities must be to a degree appropriate to the magnitude of problems and commensurate with the risks encountered.

The manufacturer must implement and record any changes to the documented procedures resulting from corrective and preventive action.

7.14.2.2 Corrective Action

The procedures for corrective action must include:

- the effective handling of customer complaints and reports of product noncomformities
- investigation of the cause of noncomformities relating to product, process, and quality management system, and recording the results of the investigation
- determination of the corrective action needed to eliminate the cause of the nonconformities
- application of controls to ensure that corrective action is taken and that it is effective.

7.14.2.3 Preventive Action

The procedures for preventive action must include:

- the use of appropriate sources of information such as processes and work operations which affect product quality, concessions, audit results, quality records, service reports, and customer complaints to detect, analyze, and eliminate potential causes of nonconformities
- determination of the steps needed to deal with any problems requiring preventive action
- initiation of preventive action and application of controls to ensure that it is effective
- confirmation that relevant information on actions taken is submitted for management review.

7.15 Handling, Storage, Packaging, Preservation, and Delivery

7.15.1 Requirements

This clause has the following requirements:

- Procedures must be established and maintained for handling, storage, packaging, preservation, and delivery of product
- Handling methods must prevent damage or deterioration
- Storage areas must be used to prevent damage or deterioration of product
- Packing, packaging, and marking processes must be controlled to the extent necessary to ensure conformance to specified requirements
- Appropriate methods for preservation and segregation of product must be applied
- Protection of the quality of the product after final inspection and test must be arranged, including delivery to its destination.

7.15.2 Compliance

7.15.2.1 Procedures

Documented procedures must be established and maintained for handling, storage, packaging, preservation, and delivery of product.

7.15.2.2 Handling

Methods of handling product that prevent damage or detioration must be established and maintained.

7.15.2.3 Storage

Designated storage areas or stock rooms must be used to prevent damage or deterioration of product, pending use or delivery. Appropriate methods for authorizing receipt to and dispatch from such areas must be stipulated. In addition, the condition of product in stock must be assessed at appropriate intervals in order to assess deterioration.

Suitable storage procedures should take into account:

- physical security
- environmental control, including temperature and humidity
- periodic checking to detect deterioration

- legible, durable marking and labeling methods
- expiration dates and stock rotation methods.

7.15.2.4 Packaging

The manufacturer must control packing, packaging, and marking processes to the extent necessary to ensure conformance to specified requirements. Packaging procedures should:

- provide appropriate protection against damage, deterioration, or contamination as long as the material remains the responsibility of the supplier
- provide a clear description of the contents or ingredients, according to regulations or to the contract
- provide for checking packaging effectiveness.

7.15.2.5 Preservation

The manufacturer must apply appropriate methods for preservation and segregation of product when the product is under the manufacturer's control.

7.15.2.6 Delivery

Protection of the quality of the product must be ensured after final protection and test. Where specified in a contract, this protection must be extended to include delivery to destination.

7.16 Control of Quality Records

7.16.1 Requirements

This clause has the following requirements:

- Procedures must be established and maintained for identification, collection, indexing, access, filing, storage, maintenance, and disposition of quality records
- Quality records must be maintained to demonstrate conformance to specified requirements and the effective operation of the quality system
- All quality records must be legible
- All quality records must be stored and retained in such a way that they are readily retrievable

- All quality records must be stored in an environment that prevents damage or deterioration and prevents loss
- Retention times of quality records must be established and recorded
- Where agreed contractually, quality records must be made available for evaluation by the customer or the customer's representative for an agreed period.

7.16.2 Compliance

7.16.2.1 Procedures

Documented procedures must be established and maintained for identification, collection, indexing, access, filing, storage, maintenance, and disposition of quality records. Such procedures should ensure records are:

- legible and identifiable to the product involved
- stored/maintained such that they are readily retrievable
- kept in an environment that prevents deterioration or damage.

7.16.2.2 Records

Quality records must be maintained to demonstrate conformance to specified requirements and the effective operation of the quality management system. Pertinent quality records from vendors must be an element of this data. Records may be in the form of any type of media, such as hard copy or electronic media.

7.16.2.3 Retention Times

Retention times must be established and recorded. Where required in the contract, quality records must be made available for evaluation by the customer or the customer's representative for an agreed time period. The following should be considered in specifying a minimum time period for retaining quality records:

- the requirements of regulatory authorities
- product liability and other legal issues related to record keeping

- the expected lifetime of the product
- the requirements of the contract.

7.17 Internal Quality Audits

7.17.1 Requirements

This clause has the following requirements:

- Procedures must be established and maintained for planning and implementing internal quality audits
- Internal quality audits must be scheduled on the basis of the status and importance of the activity to be audited
- Internal quality audits must be carried out by personnel independent of those having direct responsibility for the activity being audited
- The results of audits must be documented and brought to the attention of the personnel having responsibility in the area audited
- Management personnel responsible for the audited area must take timely corrective action on deficiencies found during the audit
- Follow-up audit activities must verify and record the implementation and effectiveness of the corrective action taken.

7.17.2 Compliance

7.17.2.1 Audit Procedures

Documented procedures must be established and maintained for planning and implementing internal quality audits to verify whether quality activities and related results comply with planned arrangements and to determine the effectiveness of the quality management system.

7.17.2.2 Audit Schedules

Internal quality audits must be scheduled on the basis of the status and importance of the activity to be audited. They must be carried out by personnel independent of those having direct responsibility for the activity being audited.

7.17.2.3 Audit Results

The results of audits must be recorded and brought to the attention of the personnel having responsibility in the area audited. Management personnel responsible for the area must take timely corrective action on deficiencies found during the audit. Follow-up audit activities must verify and record the implementation and effectiveness of the corrective action taken.

Internal audit results should form an integral part of the input to management review activities.

7.18 Training

7.18.1 Requirements

Training has the following requirements:

- Procedures must be established and maintained for identifying training needs and provide for the training of all personnel performing activities affecting quality
- Personnel performing specific assigned tasks must be qualified on the basis of appropriate education, training, and/or experience.

7.18.2 Compliance

7.18.2.1 Procedures

Documented procedures must be established and maintained for identifying training needs. They must provide for the training of all personnel performing activities affecting quality. Personnel performing specific assigned tasks must be qualified on the basis of appropriate education, training, and/or experience, as required. The training process should include:

- evaluation of the education and experience of personnel
- identification of individual training needs
- provision for appropriate training, either in-house or by external bodies

- records of training progress and updates to identify training needs.

7.18.2.2 Records

Appropriate records of training must be established and maintained. Training records should include:

- name of the individual
- identification of the training
- purpose of the training
- date the training took place
- location the training took place
- agenda of the training program.

A copy of a certificate of completion should also be placed in the individual's training record.

7.19 Servicing

7.19.1 Requirements

Servicing has the following requirements:

- Where servicing is a specified requirement, procedures must be established and maintained for performing, verifying, and reporting that the servicing meets the specified requirements.

7.19.2 Compliance

7.19.2.1 Procedures

Documented procedures must be established and maintained for performing, verifying, and reporting that the servicing meets the specified requirements. This includes:

- establishing and maintaining documented procedures for servicing, when required by the contract
- verifying and reporting that servicing meets specified requirements
- clarifying servicing responsibilities
- planning service activities
- validating the design and function of necessary servicing tools and equipment
- controlling measuring and test equipment
- providing suitable documentation and instructions
- providing backup technical advice, support and spares or parts supply
- providing competent, trained service personnel
- gathering useful feedback for product or servicing design.

7.20 Statistical Techniques

7.20.1 Requirements

Statistical techniques has the following requirements:

- The need for statistical techniques for establishing, controlling, and verifying process capability and product characteristics must be identified
- Procedures must be established and maintained to implement and control the application of statistical techniques.

7.20.2 Compliance

7.20.2.1 Procedures

The need for statistical techniques required for establishing, controlling, and verifying process capability and product characteristics must be identified. Where the need exists, documented procedures must be established and maintained to implement and control the application of these statistical techniques.

The application of statistical methods may include:

- market analysis
- product design
- reliability specifications, longevity/durability predictions
- process control/process capability studies
- determination of quality levels/inspection plans
- data analysis/performance assessment/defect analysis
- process improvement
- safety evaluation and risk analysis.

Statistical methods may include:

- graphical methods to help diagnose problems
- statistical control charts to monitor and control production measurement processes
- experiments to identify and quantify variables that influence process and product performance
- regression analysis to provide quantitative models for a process
- analysis of variance methods.

References

Fries, Richard C., *Reliable Design of Medical Devices.* New York: Marcel Dekker, Inc., 1997.

International Organization for Standardization, *ISO 9001*. Geneva: International Organization for Standardization, 1994.

Chapter 8

The ISO 14000 Series of Standards

Continual quality improvement has become a prerequisite for competitiveness. It is clear that in the future, environmental awareness combined with public and government pressure will move environmental management in the same direction. One of the most visible ways for an organization to demonstrate that it takes environmental management seriously is to implement an internationally recognized environmental-management- system standard such as the ISO 14000 series and then to have its compliance confirmed by an independent third party.

The decision to implement and register such a system, however, is not to be taken lightly. Some of the most common concerns and questions involve cost, the bottom line, the advantage of third-party assessment, and the integration of environmental and quality systems. The answers to these questions are sometimes confusing.

8.1 History of ISO 14000

ISO formed Technical Committee (TC) 207 in 1993 to develop standards in the field of environmental management tools and systems. The work of negotiating and drafting the specific standards is carried out by subcommittees. Individuals developing standards within the ISO represent private- and public-sector representatives from countries around the world. Each country is represented in the ISO by an organization which serves as the ISO member body. In the U.S., this body is the American National Standard Institute (ANSI).

Currently the ISO/TC 207 TAG has about 600 members who share a commitment and an understanding: you either help make the standards or play the game by your competitor's rules. More than 500 representatives from 47 international delegations attended the Oslo TC 207 plenary, the largest attendance ever for TC 207 and an indicator of the mounting interest generated worldwide. At these meetings, the delegates also elevated the EMS guidance standard (ISO 14004) and three auditing standards to DIS status as well. Meanwhile, work progressed on the other 14000 series life-cycle assessment, environmental labeling standards.

The work of ISO/TC 207 encompasses seven areas:

management systems
audits
labeling
environmental performance evaluation
life-cycle assessment
terms and definitions
environmental aspects in product standards.

The ISO 14000 standards are not product standards, nor do they specify performance or pollutant/effluent levels. They specifically exclude test methods for pollutants and do not set limit values regarding pollutants or effleunts.

According to TC 207 guiding principles, the 14000 standards are intended to promote the broad interests of the public and users, be cost effective, non-prescriptive and flexible, and be more easily accepted and implemented. The goal is to improve environmental protection and quality of life.

The many environmental management standards, various eco-labeling regulations and programs, and diverse life-cycle methodologies that have been established across the globe are potential trade barriers that ISO 14000 standards seek to resolve. They also may provide a reasonable alternative to traditional government command and control regulation.

The ISO 14001 environmental management standard was published in

September, 1996. Similar in structure to ISO 9000, ISO 14000 is based on the popular Deming model of management, with the key ingredients being:

PLAN
DO
CHECK
ACT.

8.2 Purpose

ISO 14001 specifies requirements for an environmental management system to enable an organization to formulate a policy and objectives taking into account legislative requirements and information about significant environmental impacts. It applies to those environmental aspects which the organization can control and over which it can be expected to have an influence. It does not state specific performance criteria.

The standard is applicable to any organization that wishes to:

implement, maintain and improve an environmental management system,

ensure itself of its conformance with its stated environmental policy,

demonstrate such conformance to others,

seek certification/registration of its environmental management system by an external organization,

make a self-determination and self-declaration of conformance with this standard.

All the requirements in this standard are intended to be incorporated into any environmental management system. The extent of the application will depend on such factors as the environmental policy of the organization, the nature of its activities, and the conditions in which it operates.

8.3 The ISO 14000 Series of Standards

The 14000 Series of Standards is composed of the following documents:

ISO 14001	Environmental Management Systems - Specification with Guidance for Use
ISO 14004	Environmental Management Systems - General Guidelines on Principles, Systems, and Supporting Techniques
ISO 14010	Guidelines for Environmental Auditing - General Principles
ISO 14011	Guidelines for Environmental Auditing - Audit Procedures - Auditing of Environmental Management Systems
ISO 14012	Guidelines for Environmental Auditing - Qualification Criteria for Environmental Auditors

8.4 14001

ISO 14001 is the basic standard for the 14000 series on the environment. It is a specification document. To be 14001 registered, an organization will have to demonstrate its environmental management system meets all the specified criteria, including:

policy and planning
organizational structure and responsibilities
training
communications
documentation
auditing
periodic management review.

8.5 Why Certify to ISO 14001?

Although national environmental management standards and industry environmental codes of practice have proliferated in recent years, an international environmental management standard offers a number of advantages to domestic and multinational companies alike. As is true for all ISO standards, the creation of ISO 14001 was through consensus of interested parties from nearly 50 countries. Delegates and experts were guided by the following concepts.

A standard that is unduly burdensome defeats two major benefits of standardization: simplicity and reduced cost. Rather than providing something completely new, ISO 14001 reflects the best practices that exist in a variety of settings. The elements incorporate components that are found in a number of standards and codes of practice.

Public disclosure is an internal management decision to be made by individual companies. Conformity to ISO 14001 does not empower individual stakeholders, organizations, or other external interested parties with the right to obtain sensitive information. Requiring such disclosure is outside the purview of the standard and does not further ISO's goal of improving environmental management.

ISO standards are not intended to serve as substitutes for or supplements to national laws and regulations. Therefore, ISO 14001 does not establish specific performance levels and rates of improvement. The standard provides a framework that allows individual companies the latitude to establish their own policies and performance objectives.

Third party verification of conformity to the standard is not required. Organizations have the option to self-audit and self-declare the adoption of ISO 14001.

8.6 Benefits of ISO 14001

The benefits of implementing ISO 14001 are as varied as the organizations that have elected to conform to the standard. The nature of a company's operations, the regulations with which it must comply, its traditional approach to addressing changing customer demands, emerging technologies, and capital investments will influence the areas in which the greatest benefits are derived. The most significant benefits fall into six areas:

- assurance of policy implementation

- worldwide consistency for multinational companies
- customer satisfaction
- reduced costs
- improved public image
- improved relations with regulatory agencies.

8.6.1 Assurance of Policy Implementation

Many companies have had the experience of devoting time and resources to the development of an environmental policy and displaying it where it will be seen by visitors and guests, only to discover that it has little effect on the way in which various operating units function on a day-to-day basis. ISO 14001 forces organizations to overcome inertia by linking the policy to articulated objectives and targets.

Making the environmental policy one of the two key elements on which the environmental management system is based, yields two outcomes. First, the policy tends to be meaningful in terms of an organization's operations and activities. The need to develop objectives and targets that contribute to the achievement of the policy prevent companies from making empty promises. Second, the requirement for top management review to ascertain the possible need for changes to the environmental policy ensures that the policy will be viable despite changing company circumstances.

8.6.2 Worldwide Consistency for Multinational Companies

ISO 14001 provides a mechanism for operating in an environmentally responsible manner in locations where local standards are minimal or do not exist. ISO 14001 does not export any country's environmental management requirements to another. Rather, it provides an internally consistent approach to environmental concerns.

Implementation of ISO 14001 has the potential to distinguish companies as environmentally concerned business partners throughout the world. It is likely to be a valuable asset in working with host governments that are interested in establishing regulatory frameworks based on performance rather than prescriptive, command-and-control requirements.

8.6.3 Customer Satisfaction

There is little question that most organizations will implement ISO 14001 in response to demand from key customers. Original equipment manufacturers will be influenced strongly by the industry sectors that they serve.

8.6.4 Reduced Costs

The ISO 14001 emphasis on prevention of pollution can reduce costs in two ways: decreased expenditures on raw materials and decreased waste disposal costs. Efforts to prevent pollution encourage attention to the toxicity of materials used in operating processes and other activities. This can result in more efficient use of toxic materials or their elimination through material substitution.

When toxic materials are used more efficiently or replaced, the environmental impact of process waste streams is lessened. Less waste, in turn, results in reduced costs associated with treatment, transport, and disposal.

Costs savings also may be realized in reduced fines and/or penalties. The Environmental Protection Agency's self-policing policy, discussed in Section 8.7, provides relief under certain circumstances for organizations that have implemented an environmental management system.

8.6.5 Improved Public Image

It is difficult to quantify the impact of public perception. However, organizations have reported that local citizens and community groups react positively to the news that ISO 14001 is being implemented.

This reaction contrasts sharply with the position taken by a small number of environmental special-interest groups. Although some environmental groups support the objectives of ISO 14001, others have been critical that it does not go far enough.

8.6.6 Improved Relations with Regulatory Agencies

State departments of environmental protection have reacted to ISO 14001 with varying degrees of interest. While most states are taking a wait-and-see attitude, a small number have indicated that ISO 14001 certification has the potential to serve as a substitute for certain regulatory requirements. Equally compelling is the level of interest expressed by the Environmental Protection Agency through a variety of proposals and pilot projects.

8.7 The Environmental Protection Agency's Self-Audit Policy

In April, 1995, the Environmental Protection Agency developed an interim audit policy to provide incentives for regulated entities that conduct voluntary compliance evaluations and also disclose and correct violations. However, this policy did not favor privilege and immunity. It stated that an environmental audit privilege could be misused to shield bad companies or to frustrate access to crucial factual information.

In January, 1996, the Environmental Protection Agency's final policy on Incentives for Self-Policing went into effect. It included:

- discovery
- disclosure
- correction
- prevention of violations.

In an effort to encourage voluntary identification of violations, the Environmental Protection Agency's policy offers several incentives, including:

- elimination of gravity-based penalties
- reduction of gravity-based penalties
- no recommendations for criminal prosecution.

In order to qualify for these incentives, specified conditions must be met:

- the violation was discovered through an environmental audit or an objective, documented systematic procedure or practice
- the violation was identified voluntarily
- the regulated entity fully discloses the violation within ten days, or less if required by law, in writing to the Environmental Protection Agency

- the violation must be discovered and disclosed independent of government or third-party plaintiff
- the regulated entity corrects the violation within 60 days and certifies in writing that the violation has been corrected
- the regulated entity agrees in writing to take steps to prevent a recurrence of the violation
- the specific violation has not occurred previously within the past three years at the same facility, or is not part of a pattern of violations by the parent organization within the past five years
- the violation did not result in serious actual harm to human health or the environment or violate the specific terms of any judicial or administrative order or consent decree
- the regulated entity cooperates as requested by the Environmental Protection Agency.

Failure to fulfill these conditions means the incentives do not apply.

8.7.1 Elimination of Gravity-Based Penalties

The Environmental Protection Agency's audit policy waives gravity-based penalties for violations under two sets of conditions:

- those that are discovered through voluntary audits and promptly disclosed and corrected

- those found through documented procedures for self-policing, where the organization can demonstrate a compliance management program.

8.7.2 Reduction of Gravity-Based Penalties

For organizations that discover, disclosure, and correct violations, but do not have an effective compliance management program, gravity-based penalties will be reduced by 75 percent. The intent of this reduction is to encourage organizations to work with the Environmental Protection Agency to resolve environmental problems and begin to develop an effective compliance management program.

8.7.3 No Recommendation for Criminal Prosecution

The Environmental Protection Agency will not recommend criminal prosecution for an organization that uncovers violations through environmental audits or due diligence, and promptly discloses and expeditiously corrects those violations. The Environmental Protection Agency reserves the right to recommend prosecution for the criminal conduct of any culpable individual.

8.8 The ISO 14001 Registration Process

Registration can be thought of as a three-tiered process that is initiated when the company seeking registration submits an application to a registrar. Organizations should select a registrar with the same diligence that is applied to the acquisition of other business services. The experience of the potential registrar in the company's industry should be a primary consideration. Other factors include the registrar's reputation and that of its accrediting body, the experience of auditors assigned to the conformity assessment, and cost.

The second tier is the performance of a conformity assessment. The registrar will evaluate the organization's environmental management system to determine whether it fulfills all the requirements of ISO 14001. Such assessments generally entail a review of relevant written policies, procedures, documents, and records, followed by an on-site assessment. Non-conformities are reported to the company. Once the organization has completed corrective action, the audit team will recommend acceptance for, or denial of, registration to the registrar.

The third tier is the awarding of a certificate to the organization. It is anticipated that ISO 14001 registration will be effective for three years, at which time the organization must reregister.

8.9 The ISO 14001 Audit

The audit should be based on objectives defined by the registering organization. The scope of the audit is determined by the lead auditor in consultation with the organization. The scope describes the extent and the boundaries of the audit. The objectives and scope of the audit should be communicated to the auditee prior to the audit. Any subsequent changes to the audit scope require the agreement of the organization and the lead auditor.

At the beginning of the audit process, the lead auditor should review the organization's documentation such as environmental policy statements, programs, records, manuals, and other appropriate documentation for meeting its environmental management system requirements. Appropriate use should be made of all appropriate background information on the auditee's organization. If the documentation is judged to be inadequate to conduct the audit, the organization should be informed.

8.9.1 The Audit Plan

The audit plan is prepared by the lead auditor. It should be designed to be flexible in order to permit changes in emphasis based on information gathered during the audit, and to permit effective use of resources. The plan, if applicable, should include:

- the audit objectives and scope
- the audit criteria
- identification of the auditee's organizational and functional units to be audited
- identification of the functions and/or individuals within the auditee's organization having significant direct responsibilities regarding the auditee's environmental management system
- identification of those elements of the auditee's environmental management system that are of high audit priority
- the procedures for auditing the auditee's environmental management system elements as appropriate for the auditee's organization
- the working and reporting languages of the audit
- identification of reference documents
- the expected time and duration for major audit activities
- the dates and places where the audit is to be conducted
- identification of audit-team members
- the schedule of meetings to be held with the auditee's management
- confidentiality requirements

- report content and format, expected date of issue, and distribution of the audit report
- document retention requirements.

The audit plan is communicated to the client, the audit team members, and the auditee. The organization should review and approve the plan. If the auditee objects to any provisions in the audit plan, such objections should be made known to the lead auditor. They should be resolved between the lead auditor, the auditee, and the client before conducting the audit. Any revised audit plan must be agreed between the parties concerned before or during the audit.

8.9.2 Working Documents

The working documents required to facilitate the auditor's investigations may include:

- forms for documenting supporting audit evidence and audit findings
- procedures and checklists used for evaluating environmental management system elements
- records of meetings.

Working documentation will be maintained at least until completion of the audit. Those involving confidential or proprietary information will be suitably safeguarded by the audit team members.

8.9.3 Conducting the Audit

There will be an opening meeting. The purpose of this meeting is to:

- introduce the members of the audit team to the auditee's management
- review the scope, objectives, and audit plan and agree on the audit timetable
- provide a short summary of the methods and procedures to be used to conduct this audit

- establish the official communication links between the audit team and the auditee
- confirm that the resources and facilities needed by the audit team are available
- confirm the time and date of the closing meeting
- promote the active participation by the auditee
- review relevant site safety and emergency procedures for the audit team.

Sufficient audit evidence will be collected to be able to determine whether the auditee's environmental management system conforms to the environmental management system audit criteria. Audit evidence will be collected through interviews, examination of documents, and observation of activities and conditions. Indications of nonconformity to the environmental management system audit criteria will be recorded. Information gathered through interviews will be verified by acquiring supporting information from independent sources, such as observations, records, and results of existing measurements. Non-verifiable statements will be identified as such.

The audit team will review all of their audit evidence to determine where the environmental management system does not conform to the environmental management system audit criteria. The audit team will them ensure that audit findings of nonconformity are documented in a clear, concise manner and supported by audit evidence. Audit findings will be reviewed with the responsible auditee manager with a view of obtaining acknowledgement of the factual basis of all findings of nonconformity.

After completion of the audit evidence collection phase and prior to preparing an audit report, the audit team will hold a closing meeting with the auditee's management and those responsible for the functions that were audited. The main purpose of the meeting is to present audit findings to the auditee in such a manner as to obtain their clear understanding and acknowledgement of the factual basis of the audit findings. Disagreements will be resolved, if possible before the lead auditor issues the report. Final decisions on the significance and description of the audit findings ultimately rest with the lead auditor, although the auditee or client may still disagree with these findings.

8.9.4 The Audit Report

The audit report will be dated and signed by the lead auditor. It contains the audit findings and/or a summary thereof with reference to supporting evidence. The audit report may include the following:

- the identification of the organization audited and of the client
- the agreed objectives, scope, and plan of the audit
- the agreed criteria, including a list of reference documents against which the audit was conducted
- the period covered by the audit and the date(s) the audit was conducted
- the identification of the auditee's representatives participating in the audit
- the identification of the audit team members
- a statement of the confidential nature of the contents
- the distribution list for the audit report
- a summary of the audit process including any obstacles encountered
- audit conclusions.

The audit report is sent to the client by the lead auditor. Distribution of the audit report is determined by the client in accordance with the audit plan. The auditee will receive a copy of the audit report unless specifically excluded by the client.

All working documents and draft and final reports pertaining to the audit will be retained by agreement between the client, the lead auditor, and the auditee, and in accordance with any applicable requirements.

The audit is completed once all the activities defined in the audit plan have been conlcuded.

8.10 ISO 14000 Costs

The costs of conformity to 14001, including initial system review, system improvement, and independent third-party registration fees, will depend on the size and complexity of the organization and the merits of its current environmental management and quality systems. It has been estimated that a manufacturing plant of 3,000 to 4,000 employees will pay approximately $25,000 in external costs and $175,000 in internal costs. These are comparable to registration costs for ISO 9000. The registration process itself could take up to 18 months.

8.11 Integrating ISO 14000

To succeed in integrating systems, you must concentrate and build on what already exists, as opposed to developing large manuals and operating procedures for each management system element. Be careful not to fall into the trap of developing separate and distinct procedures for each function with no links to other facets of the management system.

ISO 14000 implementation need not be costly or present unrealistic expectations. By using the quality management system, you have in place a blueprint to build the requirements of ISO 14000, health and safety, and other management practices into the fabric of the organization in a manner that won't break the bank.

References

Block, Marilyn, *Implementing ISO 14001.* Milwaukee: ASQC Quality Press, 1997.

Donaldson, John, "U.S. Companies Gear Up for ISO 14001 Certification," in *InTech*, Volume 43, Number 5, May, 1996.

Environmental Protection Agency, "Incentives for Self-Policing: Discovery, Disclosure, Correction, and Prevention of Violations," in *Federal Register.* 60, Number 246, December 22, 1995.

Hale, Gregory, "ISO 14000 Integration Tips," in *Quality Digest.* Volume 17, Number 2, February, 1997.

ISO, *ISO 14001: Environmental Management Systems - Specification with Guidance for Use.* Geneva: International Organization for Standardization, 1996.

ISO, *ISO 14004: Environmental Management Systems - General Guidelines on Principles, Systems, and Supporting Techniques.* Geneva: International

Organization for Standardization, 1996.

ISO, *ISO 14010: Guidelines for Environmental Auditing - General Principles.* Geneva: International Organization for Standardization, 1996.

ISO, *ISO 14011: Guidelines for Environmental Auditing - Audit Procedures - Auditing of Environmental Management Systems.* Geneva: International Organization for Standardization, 1996.

ISO, *ISO 14012: Guidelines for Environmental Auditing -Qualification Criteria for Environmental Auditors.* Geneva: International Organization for Standardization, 1996.

Munn, Samantha, "ISO 14001: A Proactive Approach to Managing Your Environmental Concerns," in *Compliance Engineering.* Volume 14, Number 2, March/April, 1997.

Chapter 9

ISO 14000 Requirements/Compliance

This international standard specifies requirements for an environmental management system to enable an organization to formulate a policy and objectives, taking into account legislative requirements and information about significant environmental impacts. It applies to those environmental aspects which the organization can control and which it can be expected to have an influence. It does not itself state specific environmental performance criteria.

This standard is applicable to any organization that wishes to:

- **implement, maintain, and improve an environmental management system**
- **assure itself of its conformance with its stated environmental policy**
- **demonstrate such conformance to others**
- **seek certification/registration of its environmental management system by an external organization**
- **make a self-determination and self-declaration of conformance with this standard.**

9.1 General Requirements

9.1.1 Requirement

This clause has the following requirement:

- Management must establish and maintain an environmental management system.

9.1.2 Compliance

Implementation of an environmental management system should result in improved environmental performance. This is based on the concept that the organization will periodically review and evaluate its environmental management system in order to identify opportunities for improvement and their implementation. Improvements in its environmental management system are intended to result in additional improvements in environmental performance.

The environmental management system provides a structured process for the achievement of continual improvement, and the rate and extent of which will be determined by the organization in the light of economic and other circumstances. Although some improvement in environmental performance can be expected due to the adoption of a systematic approach, it should be understood that the environmental management system is a tool which enables the organization to achieve and systematically control the level of environmental performance that it sets itself. The establishment and operation of an environmental management system will not, in itself, necessarily result in an immediate reduction of adverse environmental impact.

An organization has the freedom and flexibility to define its boundaries and may choose to implement this standard with respect to the entire organization, or to specific operating units or activities of the organization. If this standard is implemented for a specific operating unit or activity, policies and procedures developed by other parts of the organization can be used to meet the requirements of this standard, provided they are applicable to the specific operating unit or activity that will be subject to it. The level of detail and complexity of the environmental management system, the extent of documentation and the resources devoted to it, will be dependent on the size of an organization and the nature of its activities. This may be the case in particular for small and medium-sized enterprises. Integration of environmental matters with the overall management system, as well as to efficiency and to clarity of roles.

This standard contains management system requirements based on the dynamic cyclical process of :

- plan
- implement
- check
- review.

The system should enable an organization to:

- establish an environmental policy appropriate to itself
- identify the environmental aspects arising from the organization's past, existing, or planned activities, products, or services, to determine the environmental impacts of significance
- identify the relevant legislative and regulatory requirements
- identify priorities and set appropriate environmental objectives and targets
- establish a structure and program to implement the policy and achieve objectives and targets
- facilitate planning, control, monitoring, corrective action, auditing, and review activities to ensure both that the policy is complied with and that the environmental management system remains appropriate
- be capable of adapting to changing circumstances.

9.2 Environmental Policy

9.2.1 Requirements

This clause has the following requirements:

- Management must define the organization environmental policy
- Management must ensure the policy is appropriate to the nature, scale, and environmental impacts of its activities, products, or services
- The policy must include a commitment to continual improvement and prevention of pollution

- The policy must include a commitment to comply with relevant environmental legislation and regulations, and with other requirements to which the organization subscribes
- The policy must provide the framework for setting and reviewing environmental objectives and targets
- The policy must be documented, implemented, maintained, and communicated to all empolyees
- The policy must be available to the public.

9.2.2 Compliance

The environmental policy is the driver for implementing and improving the organization's environmental management system so that it can maintain and potentially improve its environmental performance. The policy should therefore reflect the commitment of top management to compliance with applicable laws and continual improvement. The policy forms the basis upon which the organization sets its objective and targets.

The policy should be sufficiently clear to be capable of being understood by internal and external interested parties and should be periodically reviewed and revised to reflect changing conditions and information. Its area of application should be clearly identifiable.

The environmental policy is defined as:

> a statement of a company's intentions and principles in relation to its overall environmental performance, which provides a framework for establishing objectives and targets.

Typically, policy statements assert that the company will comply with all applicable laws and regulations, protect the health and safety of its employees, and safeguard the environment.

The standard also requires that the environmental policy include four specific commitments. These commitments are:

- compliance with relevant environmental legislation and regulations
- compliance with other requirements to which the organization voluntarily subscribes

- continual improvement
- prevention of pollution.

The policy must be documented. Many companies display their policies in public areas, such as the building reception area. Many distribute their policy as internal documents, such as plastic-covered cards, or screen savers on their PCs.

Management must communicate the meaning of the policy to all employees throughout the organization. This could be accomplished through new employee orientation, company newsletters, ISO 14000 training sessions, or videotapes. It is equally important to determine whether employees understand the policy. This can be assessed through internal audits or spot checks on the employees knowledge of the policy.

The environmental policy must be available to the public. At the very least, this requires some mechanism to respond to such informational requests. More proactive companies will disseminate such information to targeted constituencies, including shareholders, customers, suppliers, and regulators.

Establishing the policy and communicating it to employees is a worthwhile effort. However, it must be followed by the implementation and maintenance of the requirements within that policy. It is only when the policy is implemented and maintained in everyday activity, that management can be certain the employees really understand the meaning of the policy.

Some examples of environmental policies include:

- It is the policy of Company X to manage all phases of our operations to minimize adverse effects on the environment and the safety and health of our employees
- Company X is committed to achieving recognition as an industrial leader in employee safety and health and environmental protection.

9.3 Planning

9.3.1 Requirements

This clause has the following requirements:

- Management must establish and maintain procedures to identify the environmental aspects of its activities, products, and services that it can control and over which it can be expected to have an influence, in order to determine those which have or can have significant impacts on the environment
- Management must ensure the aspects related to these significant impacts are considered in setting its environmental objectives
- Management must keep these procedures current
- Procedures must be established and maintained to identify and have access to legal and other requirements to which the organization subscribes
- Environmental objectives and targets must be established and maintained
- Programs for achieving the objectives and targets must be established and maintained.

9.3.2 Compliance

Planning encompasses four components:

- identification of environmental aspects
- understanding of legal and other requirements
- establishment of objectives and targets
- creation of an environmental management program.

All components are designed to ensure fulfillment of the environmental policy.

9.3.2.1 Identification of Environmental Aspects

An environmental aspect is any element of an organization's activities, products, or services that can interact with the environment. An environmental impact is any change in the environment as a result of the aspect. Figure 9.1 illustrates the distinction between environmental aspects and impacts for a manufacturing process, a product, and a service.

The standard requires the organization to have a procedure to identify its environmental aspects and their impacts. Those aspects associated with significant environmental impacts are to be considered in the development of objectives and targets. The typical approach to identification of environmental aspects involves examination of individual processes. During assessment to the standard, actual or potential environmental aspects and their impacts are secondary to the procedures by which such aspects are identified and their impacts evaluated.

Environmental impacts can be acute or chronic. Acute impacts are associated with episodic or short term events. Chronic impacts result from long-term events. Typically, environmental impact is assessed by estimating its likelihood and amplitude. Likelihood will vary according to the status of the operation or process under review. Therefore it should be assessed by considering:

- normal operating conditions
- start-up and shutdown conditions
- abnormal operating conditions
- emergency situations.

Amplitude expresses the more extensive the impact, the more significant the aspect.

The likelihood and amplitude of environmental impacts should be quantified. In the absence of such data, organizations often obtain information from a variety of sources, including scientific journals, regulatory and legislative monitoring, and trade and professional associations

An organization with no existing environmental management system should, initially, establish its current position with regard to the environment by means of a review. The aim should be to consider all environmental aspects of the organization as a basis for establishing the environmental management system. The review should cover four key areas:

- legislative and regulatory requirements
- an identification of significant environmental aspects
- an examination of all existing environmental management practices and procedures
- an evaluation of feedback from the investigation of previous incidents.

In all cases, consideration should be given to normal and abnormal operations within the organization, and to potential emergency conditions.

	Process	Product	Service
Example	Manufacture of acrylonitrile monomer	Styrofoam coffee cup	Lawn maintenance
Aspect	Ammonium Sulfate	Not degradable or recyclable	Application of herbicides or pesticides
Impact	Injection of ammonium sulfate into deep wells	Accumulation of cups in landfills	Non point source pollution

Figure 9.1 Examples of aspects and impacts. (From Block, 1997)

9.3.2.2 Understanding of Legal and Other Requirements

An organization should have a procedure to identify the legal requirements with which it must comply. It must also have a procedure to provide access to those requirements. This would include international, federal, state, and local laws and regulations. The procedures are likely to require periodic updating as changes are enacted. Similar procedures must be established for voluntary initiatives to which the organization subscribes. These must also be communicated to all employees.

9.3.2.3 Establishment of Objectives and Targets

Environmental objectives are overall environmental goals. Examples of objectives include:

- reduce paper usage
- reduce energy usage.

Environmental targets are detailed performance requirements that must be met to achieve environmental objectives. An example would be:

to reduce paper by 15% over the previous year's use.

The objectives should be specific and targets should be measurable wherever practicable, and where appropriate, take preventive measures into account. When considering their technological options, an organization may consider the use of the best available technology where economically viable, cost-effective, and judged appropriate.

9.3.2.4 Creation of an Environmental Management Program

The creation and use of one or more programs is a key element to the successful implementation of an environmental management system. The program should describe how the organization's objectives and targets will be achieved, including time-scales and personnel responsible for implementing the organization's environmental policy. The program may be subdivided to address specific elements of the organization's operations. The program should include an environmental review for new activities.

The environmental management program is directly tied to objectives and targets. It encompasses the planning and logistics that enable an organization to achieve the targets that it has set for itself.

Some companies will integrate the environmental management program with other planning efforts, such as strategic planning. Others will find it easier to maintain the environmental management program as a separate initiative. Whether an integrated or independent approach is used, an effective program will address critical activities designed to achieve objectives and targets, departmental and individual responsibility for the implementation of those activities, resources timing, and milestones. The program should also identify the measures that will be used to track progress in achieving established targets.

9.4 Implementation and Operation

9.4.1 Requirements

This clause has the following requirements:

- Management must define, document, and communicate roles, responsibilities, and authorities
- Management must provide resources essential to the implementation and control of the environmental management system

- Management shall appoint a specific management representative(s) who has defined roles, responsibilities, and authorities.
- Management must identify training needs
- Management must ensure that all personnel whose work may create a significant impact on the environment, have received appropriate training
- Management must establish and maintain procedures to ensure personnel are aware of the importance of conformance with the environmental policy, the significant impact of the work activities, their roles and responsibilities, and the potential consequences of departure from specified procedures
- Management must ensure personnel performing the tasks causing significant environmental impact are competent, on the basis of appropriate education, training, and/or experience
- Procedures for internal communications must be established and maintained
- Procedures for receiving, documenting, and responding to relevant communication from external parties must be established and maintained
- Documentation must be established and maintained that describes the core elements of the management system and their interaction
- Documentation must be established and maintained to provide direction to related documentation
- Procedures must be established and maintained for controlling all documents required by the standard
- Documentation must be legible, dated, readily identifiable, maintained in an orderly manner, and retained for a specific period
- Procedures and responsibilities must be established and maintained concerning the creation and modification of the various types of document
- Management must identify those operations and activities that are associated with the identified significant environmental aspects in line with its policy, objectives, and targets
- Procedures must be established and maintained to identify potential for and respond to accidents and emergency

situations, and for preventing and mitigating the environmental impact that may be associated with them
- Management must review and revise, where necessary, its emergency preparedness and response procedures
- Management must periodically test its emergency preparedness and response procedures.

9.4.2 Compliance

Implementation and operation involves carrying out actions that were identified during the planning stage. This section contains seven elements that must be addressed:

- structure and responsibility
- training, awareness, and competence
- communication
- documentation
- document control
- operational control
- emergency preparedness and response.

9.4.2.1 Structure and Responsibility

The successful implementation of an environmental management system calls for the commitment of all employees of the organization. Environmental responsibilities therefore should not be seen as confined to the environmental function, but may also include other areas of an organization, such as operational management or staff functions other than environmental.

This commitment should begin at the highest levels of management. Accordingly, top management should establish the organization's environmental policy and ensure that the environmental management system is implemented. As part of this commitment, top management should designate a specific management representative with defined responsibility and authority for implementing the environmental management system. Top management should also ensure that appropriate resources are provided to ensure that the environmental management system is implemented and maintained. It is also important that the key environmental management system responsibilities are well defined and communicated to the relevant personnel.

The distinction between responsibility and authority is important for understanding the intended purpose of this element. Within the context of an environmental management system, responsibility pertains to specific tasks or obligations with which one is charged. Authority pertains to influence and power. An individual with responsibility does not necessarily have authority. The standard attempts to ensure that a chief environmental officer has the power to guarantee that assigned responsibilities are accomplished and needed resources are available to fulfill requirements.

9.4.2.2 Training, Awareness, and Competence

The organization should establish and maintain procedures for identifying training needs. The organization should also require that contractors working on its behalf are able to demonstrate that their employees have the requisite training.

Management should determine the level of experience, competence, and training necessary to ensure the capability of personnel, especially those carrying out specialized environmental management functions.

This element addresses to areas of training:

- skills or competence training for employees whose work may have a significant environmental impact
- general awareness training for employees throughout the organization.

Personnel whose work can cause significant environmental impact must be competent to perform those tasks. Competence, defined as the effective execution of required actions, can be attained through avenues other than training, such as formal education and/or experience. It is incumbent upon management to define competence and identify training needs for those employees whose on-the-job performance does not meet defined competence levels. It quickly becomes apparent that identification of training needs is directly related to identification of a company's environmental aspects and their significant environmental impacts. Therefore, training needs are likely to go beyond those courses that are mandated by regulations.

General awareness training is intended to emphasize the importance of conforming to the standard and reinforce the environmental benefits of improved individual performance. Therefore, such training should be offered to a broad array of employees, at all levels, from senior management to the most junior individuals in the organization. It should be designed to fulfill the following objectives:

- make all employees aware of the company's commitment to be the environmental leader in its industry
- create awareness of each employee's individual environmental responsibilities
- create a behavior change that will improve employees environmental performance.

All training must be documented. This will help fulfill the requirements in the records section as well.

9.4.2.3 Communication

Many companies have far-reaching communication mechanisms that cascade information down through the organization. Less pervasive are procedures for encouraging communication across functional areas and from lower levels up to higher levels in the organization. As used in the requirements, *relevant level and function* refers to multidirectional internal communication procedures that enable access to relevant information.

The standard does not require public disclosure of any other environmental information other than the environmental policy. The only communication requirement applicable to external parties is reactive in nature. Organizations must document and respond to relevant communication.

9.4.2.4 Documentation

Documentation of the environmental management system can take any form that is useful to an organization. The standard does not require a single manual, nor does it dictate the kinds of information that should be maintained. However, organizations that have or are in the process of obtaining ISO 9000 certification will benefit from the ability to easily integrate the two sets of documentation. Related documentation may include:

- process information

- organizational charts
- internal and operational procedures
- site emergency plans.

The level of detail of the documentation should be sufficient to describe the core elements of the environmental management system and their interaction and provide direction on where to obtain more detailed information on the operation of specific parts of the environmental management system.

Environmental management system documentation, based on the ISO 9000 model, will encompass the following three levels:

- an environmental management system manual
- environmental management system procedures
- environmental records, reports, forms, and other similar accounts and measure of environmental performance.

Some companies may elect to expand their documentation by including work instructions. These detailed explanations of how specific tasks are to be carried out should reflect the organization's environmental aspects and regulatory requirements.

9.4.2.5 Document Control

The purpose of this requirement is to ensure that organizations create and maintain documents in a manner sufficient to implement the environmental management system. According to the standard, three procedures must be documented:

- operating procedures for activities associated with significant aspects
- monitoring and measurement of activities that can have a significant environmental impact
- periodic evaluation of regulatory compliance.

In addition, eleven activities must be documented:

- environmental policy
- environmental objectives

- roles, responsibilities, and authorities
- communication from external parties
- decisions regarding external communication about significant environmental aspects
- environmental management system documentation
- calibration and maintenance of monitoring equipment
- changes in any documentation procedures
- training
- results of audits and reviews
- management review of the environmental management system.

Another eleven elements require that the organization establish and maintain procedures without requiring that such procedures be documented:

- identification of environmental aspects
- identification of and access to legal and other requirements
- identification of training needs
- internal communication
- receiving, documenting, and responding to relevant communication from external interested parties
- document control
- identifiable significant environmental aspects of goods and services used by the organization
- identification of the potential for and response to accidents and emergencies
- defining responsibility and authority for addressing non-conformance and corrective/preventive action
- identification, maintenance, and disposition of environmental records
- environmental management system audits.

The organization must establish a procedure for managing all of its documents. All documentation should be clear, usable, and informative. If it is not understandable either by those within the organization or external auditors, it is not useful.

Documentation may appear on paper or in electronic form. Flowcharts may supplement or replace text. Organizations should use whatever mechanisms and formats contribute most effectively to the utility of the document in question.

9.4.2.6 Operational Control

Most companies have documented operating procedures and work instructions for every facet of their operations. Many of these procedures and instructions implicitly address environmental concerns. The standard does not require documented procedures for every activity associated with significant environmental aspects. It requires such procedures for those activities where the lack of a procedure could result in a failure to adequately address established environmental priorities.

9.4.2.7 Emergency Preparedness and Response

The purpose of this requirement is to ensure that organizations will respond appropriately when faced with an accident or other unexpected incident. Because a comprehensive assessment of environmental aspects addresses the likelihood of environmental impact under abnormal operating conditions and emergency situations, many companies find it practical to link that procedure with this requirement. The emergency plans that are legally required in many United States companies are generally adequate to fulfill this requirement.

9.5 Checking and Corrective Action

9.5.1 Requirements

This clause has the following requirements:

- Procedures must be established and maintained to monitor and measure, on a regular basis, the key characteristics of its operations and activities that can have a significant impact on the environment.
- Monitoring equipment must be calibrated and maintained and records of this process must be retained according to the organization's procedures.
- A procedure for periodically evaluating compliance with relevant environmental legislation and regulations must be established and maintained.
- Procedures must be established and maintained for

defining responsibility and authority for handling and investigating nonconformance, taking action to mitigate any impacts caused, and for initiating and completing corrective and preventive action.

- Corrective or preventive action must be appropriate to the magnitude of problems and commensurate with the environmental impact encountered.
- Changes in the documented procedures resulting from corrective or preventive action must be implemented and recorded.
- Procedures must be established and maintained for the identification, maintenance, and disposition of environmental records.
- Environmental records must be legible, identifiable, and traceable to the activity, product, or service involved.
- Environmental records must be stored and maintained in such a way that they are readily retrievable and protected against damage, deterioration, or loss.
- Retention times for environmental records must be established and recorded.
- Programs and procedures must be established and maintained for periodic environmental management system audits to be carried out.

9.5.2 Compliance

Checking and corrective action contains four elements that are intended to measure and evaluate the effects of actions taken during implementation and operation:

- monitoring and measurement
- nonconformance and corrective and preventive action
- records
- the environmental management system audit.

9.5.2.1 Monitoring and Measurement

Organizations must compare their actual environmental performance with the performance levels designated by objectives and targets. Such comparisons are intended to determine whether the organization is achieving the goals embodied in its environmental policy and addressed through it environmental management program.

Although specific performance measurements will reflect critical environmental aspects of a company's activities and, therefore, are likely to differ from one organization to another, all performance measures should be characterized by:

- *Access* - data should be readily obtainable
- *Adequacy* - data should be appropriate for their intended use
- *Validity* - data should measure what they are intended to measure
- *Reliability* - data is accurate.

There must also be a documented procedure to determine whether the organization is in compliance with its legal requirements.

9.5.2.2 Nonconformance and Corrective and Preventive Action

This element pertains to any failure to fulfill a requirement of the standard. It does not refer to regulatory noncompliance, although it frequently is misinterpreted as such. In practice, an environmental management system audit will seek to identify nonconformities with any requirement of the standard. Therefore, nonconformances that are identified in conjunction with any assessment, audit, or other review of the environmental management system are subject to the procedures established here.

When establishing and maintaining procedures for investigating and correcting nonconformances, the cause should be identified, corrective action should be identified and implemented, controls should be implemented or modified to avoid repetition, and any changes in written procedures resulting from the corrective action should be recorded.

9.5.2.3 Records

Procedures for identification, maintenance, and disposition of records should focus on those records needed for the implementation and operation of the environmental management system and for recording the extent to which planned objectives and targets have been met. Environmental records may include:

- information on applicable environmental laws or other requirements
- complaint records
- training records
- process information
- product information
- inspection, maintenance, and calibration records
- pertinent contractor and supplier information
- incident reports
- information on emergency preparedness and response
- information on significant environmental aspects
- audit results
- management reviews.

Proper account should be taken of confidential business information.

Unless required by law, organizations are free to determine how long such records are to be maintained.

9.5.2.4 The Environmental Management System Audit

The audit program and procedures should address:

- the activities and areas to be considered in audits
- the frequency of audits
- the responsibilities associated with managing and conducting audits
- the communication of audit results
- auditor competence
- how audits will be conducted.

Audits may be performed by personnel from within the organization and/or by external persons selected by the organization. In either case, the persons conducting the audit should be in a position to do so impartially and objectively.

9.6 Management Review

9.6.1 Requirements

Management review has the following requirements:

- Management must, at intervals that it determines, review the environmental management system, to ensure its continuing suitability, adequacy, and effectiveness.
- The management review must be documented.
- The management review must address the possible need for changes to policy, objectives, and other elements of the environmental management system, due to environmental management system audit results, changing circumstances, and the commitment to continual improvement.

9.6.2 Compliance

In order to maintain continual improvement, suitability, and effectiveness of the environmental management system, and thereby its performance, the organization's management should review and evaluate the environmental management system at defined intervals. The scope of the review should be comprehensive, though not all elements of an environmental management system need to be reviewed at once and the review process may take place over a period of time.

The review of the policy, objectives, and procedures should be carried out by the level of management that defined them.

Reviews should include:

- results from audits
- the extent to which objectives and targets have been met
- the continuing suitability of the environmental management system in relation to changing conditions and information
- concerns among relevant interested parties.

Observations, conclusions, and recommendations should be documented for necessary action.

References

ANSI/ISO 14001, *Environmental Management Systems - Specification with Guidance for Use.* Geneva: International Organization for Standardization, 1996.

Block, Marilyn, *Implementing ISO 14001.* Milwaukee: ASQC Quality Press,1997.

Section 3

Quality Devices

Chapter 10

EN 46001

This standard is the current European Norm that addresses the quality system requirements for the design/development, production, and where relevant, installation and servicing of medical devices. It is used in conjunction with ISO 9001. Medical companies seeking certification to ISO 9001 usually become certified to EN 46001 at the same time.

10.1 History of EN 46001

EN 46001 was approved by CEN/CENELEC on October 22, 1993. It was prepared by the joint CEN/CENELEC Coordinating Working Group on Quality Supplements with the cooperation of CEN technical committee 205 and CENELEC technical committee 62, CENELEC technical committee 140, and the joint CEN/CENELEC Working Group on active implantable medical devices.

10.2 Scope

The standard specifies, in conjunction with ISO 9001, the quality system requirements for the design/development, production, and where relevant, installation and servicing of medical devices. This standard is used when a medical device manufacturer's quality system is assessed in accordance with regulatory requirements. As part of an assessment by a third party for the purpose of regulatory requirements, the manufacturer may be required to provide access to confidential data in order to demonstrate compliance with this standard. The manufacturer may be required to exhibit this data, but is not obliged to provide copies for retention.

10.3 Types of Medical Devices

The standard addresses several groups of medical devices. The groups are as follows:

- general medical device
- active medical device
- active implantable medical device
- implantable medical device
- in vitro diagnostic device
- non-active medical device.

The general medical device is defined as any instrument, apparatus, appliance, material, or other article, whether used alone or in combination, including the software necessary for its proper application, intended by the manufacturer for human use for the purpose of:

- diagnosis, prevention, monitoring, treatment, or alleviation of disease
- diagnosis, monitoring, treatment, or alleviation of or compensation for an injury or handicap
- investigation, replacement, or modification of the anatomy or of a physiological process
- control of conception

and which does not achieve its principal intended action in or on the human body by pharmacological, immunological, or metabolic means, but which may be assisted in its function by such means.

An active medical device is defined as any medical device relying for its functioning on a source of electrical energy or any source of power other than that directly generated by the human body or gravity.

An active implantable medical device is any active medical device which is intended to be totally or partially introduced, surgically or medically, into the human body or by medical instrumentation into a natural orifice, and which is intended to remain after the procedure.

An implantable medical device is any medical device intended:

- to be totally or partially introduced into the human body or a natural orifice, or
- to replace an epithelial surface or the surface of the eye,

by surgical intervention, which is intended to remain after the procedure for at least 30 days and which can only be removed by medical or surgical intervention.

An in vitro diagnostic device is any device which is a reagent, reagent product, kit, instrument, equipment, or system, whether used alone or in combination, intended by the manufacturer to be used in vitro for the examination of samples derived from the human body with a view to providing information on the physiological state, state of health, disease, or congenital abnormality thereof.

A non-active medical device is any medical device which is neither an active medical device nor an in vitro diagnostic device.

10.4 General Provisions

The standard follows the format of ISO 9001, listing the twenty clauses and adding requirements specifically for medical devices. Where no additional requirements for medical devices are necessary, the requirement states that the requirements of ISO 9001 shall apply.

References

European Committee for Standardization and the European Committee for Electrotechnical Standardization, *EN 46001 Quality Systems - Medical devices - Particular requirements for the application of EN 29001.* Brussels, 1993.

Chapter 11

EN 46001 Requirements/Compliance

En 46001 provides particular requirements on quality systems for suppliers of medical devices that are more specific that the general requirements specified in ISO 9001. In conjunction with ISO 9001, EN 46001 defines requirements for quality systems relating to the design/development, production, installation, and servicing of medical devices. It embraces all the principles of good manufacturing practice widely used in the manufacture of medical devices.

11.1 Management Responsibility

11.1.1 Requirements

All requirements of ISO 9001 apply The following is a particular requirement for medical devices:

Clause 4.1.2.1 The manufacturer must document the responsibility, authority, and the interrelationship of all personnel who manage, perform, and verify work affecting quality.

11.1.2 Compliance

Management must develop and maintain a document that indicates the names and authority of individuals who manage, perform, and verify quality work. The document should also contain the interrelationships of these individuals to each other and the work. The document could be as simple as a list of names and job titles. The job descriptions for the job titles could explain in detail the functions of the position.

11.2 Quality System

11.2.1 Requirements

All requirements of ISO 9001 apply. The following is a particular requirement for medical devices:

Clause 4.2.1	The manufacturer must establish and document the specified requirements.
Clause 4.2.3	The manufacturer must establish and maintain a file containing documents defining the product specifications, including complete manufacturing and quality assurance specifications for each type/model of medical device or referring to the location of this information.

11.2.2 Compliance

The manufacturer must develop and maintain a document which contains the specified requirements for a particular product. The requirements must be developed from customer and market input. The requirements document should be placed under revision control in order to track changes.

A project file or design history file must be developed for each device. The file must contain all the appropriate documents that define the requirements of the device, detail the design and development of the device, and the manufacturing and quality assurance specifications. The file may be hard copy or electronic in nature. When both exist, references to documents in the hard copy file should be made in the electronic file and vice versa. The file must be controlled. An index for the file is helpful in determining the location of specific documents within the file.

11.3 Contract Review

11.3.1 Requirements

All requirements of ISO 9001 apply.

11.3.2 Compliance

Compliance is as discussed in Section 7.3.2.

11.4 Design Control

11.4.1 Requirements

All requirements of ISO 9001 apply. The following is a particular requirement for medical devices:

Clause 4.4.3	The manufacturer must identify requirements that are related to the safety of the medical device and must include such requirements as design input data.
Clause 4.4.5	The manufacturer must document and maintain records of all design verification activities including those where clinical investigation was involved.

11.4.2 Compliance

Requirements that are related to the safety of the device must be included in the product and design specifications. These requirements will serve as a starting point for risk analysis and risk management.

All design verification activities, including clinical investigations, must be documented and placed in the project file. Documents should include:

- activity protocol
- details of the activity

- summary of the results of the activity.

Where regression testing is necessary to verify changes to the design, based on initial verification failures, documents indicating the protocol, details, and results of the regression testing must be developed and placed in the project file. Reference should be made to the initial testing which caused the subsequent testing.

11.5 Document and Data Control

11.5.1 Requirements

All requirements of ISO 9001 apply. The following is a particular requirement for medical devices:

Clause 4.5.2 — The manufacturer must define the period for which at least one copy of obsolete documents will be retained. This period must ensure that specifications to which medical devices have been manufactured are available for at least the lifetime of the medical device, as defined by the manufacturer.

11.5.2 Compliance

The manufacturer must keep the appropriate design documentation for each revision of a device for a specified period of time. This time period must be, at a minimum, the time the particular revision may exist in the field and be subject to maintenance by representatives of the manufacturer or a third party service organization. This time period must be defined and listed in a document specifically addressing maintenance of obsolete documents.

11.6 Purchasing

11.6.1 Requirements

All requirements of ISO 9001 apply. The following is a particular requirement for medical devices:

Clause 4.6.3 To the extent required by the particular requirements for traceability in Clause 4.8, the manufacturer must retain copies of relevant purchasing documents.

11.6.2 Compliance

Purchasing documents must be maintained for a period of time specified in a document addressing maintenance of design documentation. This time period should, at a minimum, be as long as a device containing the particular purchased component or assembly is active in the field and potentially subject to regulatory or legal activity.

11.7 Control of Customer-Supplied Product

11.7.1 Requirements

All requirements of ISO 9001 apply.

11.7.2 Compliance

Compliance is as discussed in Section 7.7.2.

11.8 Product Identification and Traceability

11.8.1 Requirements

All requirements of ISO 9001 apply. The following is a particular requirement for medical devices:

Clause 4.8 The manufacturer must establish and maintain procedures to ensure that medical devices received for refurbishing are identified and distinguished at all times from normal production.

> The manufacturer must establish, document, and maintain procedures for traceability. The procedures shall define the extent of traceability and facilitate corrective action.
>
> For active implantable and implantable medical devices, the extent of traceability must include all components and materials used and records of the environmental conditions when these could cause the medical device not to satisfy its specified requirements.

11.8.2 Compliance

The manufacturer must develop and maintain documentation that describes the process of refurbishing medical devices. The documents must include the requirement to keep all refurbished devices physically separate from regularly manufactured devices, to avoid the possibility of shipping a refurbished device as new.

The manufacturer must develop and maintain documentation that describes the process of traceability for its medical devices. The documentation shall address the level of assembly within the device that will be traceable. It must also detail a corrective action plan for any nonconformity within that level.

For manufacturers of active implantable and implantable medical devices, the traceability documentation must address all components and materials used within the device and the environmental conditions in which the device was manufactured when these conditions could potentially cause the device not to meet its specified requirements.

11.9 Process Control

11.9.1 Requirements

All requirements of ISO 9001 apply. The following is a particular requirement for medical devices:

<u>Clause 4.9</u>

The manufacturer must establish, document, and maintain requirements for health, cleanliness, and clothing of personnel if contact between such personnel and product or environment could adversely affect the quality of product.

The manufacturer must ensure that all personnel who are required to work temporarily under special environmental conditions are appropriately trained or supervised by a trained person.

For medical devices:

- that are supplied sterile
- that are supplied non-sterile and intended for sterilization before use
- where the microbiological and/or particulate cleanliness or other environmental conditions are of significance in their use
- where the environmental conditions are of significance in their manufacture,

the manufacture must establish and document requirements for the environment to which product is exposed. If appropriate, the environmental conditions must be controlled and/or monitored.

The manufacturer must establish, document, and maintain requirements for cleanliness of product if:

- the product is cleaned by the manufacturer prior to sterilization and/or its use
- the product is supplied non-sterile to be subjected to a cleaning process prior to sterilization and/or its use
- the product is supplied to be used non-sterile and its cleanliness is of significance in use, or

If appropriate, the product cleaned in accordance with the first or second bullet point above need not be subject to the preceding particular requirements prior to the cleaning procedure.

The manufacturer must establish and document requirements for maintenance activities when such activities may affect product quality. Records of such maintenance must be kept.

If appropriate, the manufacturer must establish and document both instructions and acceptance criteria for installing and checking the medical device. Records of installation and checking performed by the manufacturer or their authorized representative must be retained. If the contract allows installation other than by the manufacturer or their authorized representative, the manufacturer must provide the purchaser with written instructions for installation and checking.

<u>Clause 4.9.2</u> The manufacturer must ensure that the quality records identify:

- the work instruction used
- the date the special process was performed
- the identity of the operator of the special process.

For sterile medical devices, the manufacturer must subject the medical devices to a validated sterilization process and record all the control parameters of the sterilization process.

11.9.2 Compliance

The manufacturer must establish and maintain documentation detailing requirements for health, cleanliness, and personal clothing to be used during manufacturing, where contact between such personnel and the product and/or environment could adversely affect the quality of the product. These procedures are especially important with regard to such areas as clean rooms and areas sensitive to electrostatic discharge.

All personnel working under special environmental conditions or performing special processes and/or functions must be properly trained to successfully operate under those conditions, or be supervised by an individual who has been trained. The training for these individuals must be included in the individual's training record, including details of the training, date of training, and signature of the trainer.

The manufacturer must establish and maintain documentation specifying the requirements for the environment to which medical devices are exposed, including those that are supplied sterile, supplied non-sterile and intended for sterilization before use, where microbiological and/or particulate cleanliness are of significance, and where the environmental conditions are of significance during manufacture. Such procedures must include details of the methods of control of the environment and how it is to be monitored.

Procedures must be established and maintained that detail cleanliness requirements for products which are cleaned by the manufacturer prior to sterilization and/or its use, supplied non-sterile and subjected to a cleaning process prior to sterilization, supplied to be used non-sterile and its cleanliness is of significance, and where process agents are to be removed from the product during manufacture.

Procedures must be established and maintained which detail maintenance activities, where such activities affect product quality. The procedures must include a requirement for establishing and maintaining records of such maintenance, including product name, type of maintenance performed, date of maintenance, and the individual performing the work.

The manufacturer must establish and maintain detailed instructions for installing and checking each medical device. Such instructions must include or reference the acceptance criteria for the device. A record of the installation and inspection must be developed and maintained. Such record should include the device name, name of the customer, date of the installation, record of the installation instructions, any problems found during installation, and the name of the individual performing the installation.

Prior to sterilizing medical devices, the manufacturer must have validated the sterilization process and recorded the control parameters and the results of the process, including date and personnel performing the validation.

11.10 Inspection and Testing

11.10.1 Requirements

All requirements of ISO 9001 apply. The following is a particular requirement for medical devices:

Clause 4.10.4 For active implantable and implantable medical devices, the manufacturer must record the identity of personnel performing any inspection or testing.

11.10.2 Compliance

For active implantable and implantable devices, personnel performing inspection and testing must be identified. This could be accomplished directly on the inspection or test documentation by use of initials, employee number, or signature.

11.11 Control of Inspection, Measuring, and Test Equipment

11.11.1 Requirements

All requirements of ISO 9001 apply.

11.11.2 Compliance

Compliance is as discussed in Section 7.11.2.

11.12 Inspection and Test Status

11.12.1 Requirements

All requirements of ISO 9001 apply.

11.12.2 Compliance

Compliance is as discussed in Section 7.12.2.

11.13 Control of Nonconforming Product

11.13.1 Requirements

All requirements of ISO 9001 apply. The following is a particular requirement for medical devices:

<u>Clause 4.13.1</u>	The manufacturer must ensure that nonconforming product is accepted by concession only if regulatory requirements are met. The identity of the person authorizing the concession must be recorded. If the product needs to be reworked, the manufacturer must document the rework in a work instruction that has undergone the same authorization and approval procedure as the original work instruction.

11.13.2 Compliance

When concessions are developed for nonconforming product, the concession must be reviewed and approved by appropriate personnel, including the individual responsible for regulatory requirements. The concession should contain the signatures of those individuals reviewing and approving the concession.

Devices that need to be reworked must be reworked according to detailed documentation. The rework documentation must be reviewed and approved according to the same procedures used for the original work instructions.

11.14 Corrective and Preventive Action

11.14.1 Requirements

All requirements of ISO 9001 apply. The following is a particular requirement for medical devices:

Clause 4.14 — The manufacturer must establish and maintain a documented feedback system to provide early warning of quality problems and for input into the corrective action system.

If this standard is used for compliance with regulatory requirements that require post marketing surveillance, this surveillance must form part of the feedback system.

All feedback information, including reported customer complaints and returned product, must be documented, investigated, interpreted, collated, and communicated in accordance with defined procedures by a designated person.

If any customer complaint is not followed by corrective action, the rationale must be recorded.

The manufacturer must maintain records of all complaint investigations. When the investigation determines that the activities at remote premises played a part in the complaint, a copy of the report must be sent to those premises.

If this standard is used for compliance with

regulatory requirements, the manufacturer must establish, document, and maintain procedures to notify the regulatory authority of those incidents which meet the reporting criteria.

The manufacturer must establish, document, and maintain procedures for the issue of advisory notices and the recall of medical devices. These procedures must be capable of being implemented at any time.

11.14.2 Compliance

The manufacturer must establish and maintain procedures for capturing information from manufacturing and the field and providing feedback to appropriate personnel for corrective action. The procedures must detail the method of information capture, processing of the information, and feedback to appropriate personnel.

All complaints must be investigated and the appropriate corrective action taken to address the problem. If the activities at a remote site were an important part of the complaint, the site should be sent a copy of the report. Where a customer complaint is not followed by corrective action, the rationale for that action must be documented and maintained.

Procedures must be established and maintained detailing the notification of appropriate regulatory bodies when the complaint may require regulatory activity or intervention.

11.15 Handling, Storage, Packaging, Preservation, and Delivery

11.15.1 Requirements

All requirements of ISO 9001 apply. The following is a particular requirement for medical devices:

Clause 4.15.1 The manufacturer must establish and maintain documented procedures for the control of product with a limited shelf life or requiring special storage conditions. Such special storage conditions must be controlled and recorded.

If appropriate, special provisions must be made for the handling of used product in order to prevent contamination of other product, the manufacturing environment, or personnel.

<u>Clause 4.15.4</u> For sterile medical devices, the manufacturer must establish and maintain procedures to ensure that:

- the medical device is represented in a container which maintains the sterility of the medical device, except for those medical devices for which only the inner surfaces of the device are sterile and the device is such that the sterility of the inner surfaces is maintained
- the medical device is capable of being presented in an aseptic manner, if its use so requires
- the package or medical device, if only the inner surface is sterile, clearly reveals that it has been opened.

For active implantable and implantable medical devices, the manufacturer must record the identity of persons who perform the final labelling operation.

<u>Clause 4.15.5</u> For active implantable and implantable medical devices, the manufacturer must ensure that the name and address of the shipping package consignee is included in the quality records.

The manufacturer must ensure that any authorized representative maintains records of distribution of medical devices and that such records are available for inspection.

11.15.2 Compliance

Procedures must be established and maintained detailing procedures for the control of product with a limited shelf life or requiring special storage conditions. When addressing product with limited shelf life, the procedures should indicate the method of product use, such as first in, first out (FIFO).

Procedures must be established and maintained detailing special provisions for the handling or used product in order to prevent contamination of personnel, the environment, or other product. The procedure should detail how the product is to be prepared for analysis, without destroying the reason for its return.

Procedures must be established and maintained that detail the packaging and labelling of sterile medical devices. For active implantable and implantable devices, the procedure must require the identification of the individual(s) performing the final labelling operation.

For active implantable and implantable medical devices, the manufacturer must record and maintain the name and address of the shipping package consignee. These must be included in the quality records.

Records of distribution of medical devices must be established and maintained. They must be available for inspection by competent authority.

11.16 Control of Quality Records

11.16.1 Requirements

All requirements of ISO 9001 apply. The following is a particular requirement for medical devices:

Clause 4.16	The manufacturer must retain the quality records for a period of time at least equivalent to the lifetime of the medical device defined by the manufacturer, but not less than two years from the date of dispatch from the manufacturer. The manufacturer must establish and maintain a record for each batch of medical devices that

provides traceability to the extent required by clause 4.8 and identifies the quantity manufactured and quantity released for distribution. The batch record must be verified and authorized.

11.16.2 Compliance

The manufacture must develop a procedure which documents the length of time quality is to be retained and maintained. The minimum length of time for retention of the quality records must exceed two years from the date of shipment of the device.

The manufacturer must establish and maintain a record of each batch of medical devices produced. The documentation must contain traceability according to established procedures. It must also identify the quantity of devices manufactured and the quantity released for distribution. The batch record must be reviewed and signed.

11.17 Internal Quality Audits

11.17.1 Requirements

All requirements of ISO 9001 apply.

11.17.2 Compliance

The discussion is as in Section 7.17.2

11.18 Training

11.18.1 Requirements

All requirements of ISO 9001 apply. The following is a particular requirement for medical devices:

Clause 4.118 — The manufacturer must ensure that all personnel who are required to work under special environmental conditions or who perform special processes or functions are appropriately trained or supervised by a trained person.

11.18.2 Compliance

All personnel working under special environmental conditions or performing special processes and/or functions must be properly trained to successfully operate under those conditions, or be supervised by an individual who has been trained. The training for these individuals must be included in the individual's training record, including details of the training, date of training, and signature of the trainer.

11.19 Service

11.19.1 Requirements

All requirements of ISO 9001 apply.

11.19.2 Compliance

The discussion is as in Section 7.19.2

11.20 Statistical Techniques

11.20.1 Requirements

All requirements of ISO 9001 apply. The following is a particular requirement for medical devices:

Clause 4.20 — The manufacturer must establish and maintain procedures to ensure that sampling methods are regularly reviewed in the light of the occurrence of nonconforming product, quality audit reports, feedback information, and other appropriate considerations.

11.20.2 Compliance

The manufacturer must establish and maintain procedures that detail the sampling methods to be used in various parts of the development process. These documents must be reviewed on a periodic basis, taking into consideration the history of nonconforming product, quality audit reports, feedback from the field, and other sources of information regarding the functioning of the product in question.

Reference

European Committee for Standardization and the European Committee for Electrotechnical Standardization, *EN 46001 Quality Systems - Medical devices - Particular requirements for the application of EN 29001.* Brussels, 1993.

Chapter 12

The ISO 13485 Standard

This standard may be the next European Norm (EN) that addresses the quality system requirements for the design/development, production, installation, and servicing of medical devices. It can only be used in conjunction with ISO 9001:1994 and is not a stand-alone standard. It embraces all the principles of Good Manufacturing Practice widely used in the manufacture of medical devices.

12.1 History

The standard was developed by Working Group 1 of ISO Technical Committee 210. The first meeting of the Working Group was held in February, 1995. Subsequent meetings have reviewed further drafts of the document and developed it toward a European Norm.

12.2 Scope

This international standard specifies, in conjunction with ISO 9001:1994, the quality system requirements for the design/development, production, and where relevant, installation and servicing of medical devices.

This standard in conjunction with ISO 9001:1994, is applicable when there is a need to assess a medical device manufacturer's quality system or when a regulatory requirement specifies that this standard must be used for such assessment.

As part of an assessment by a third party for the purpose of regulatory requirements, the manufacturer may be required to provide access to confidential data in order to demonstrate compliance with this standard. The manufacturer may be required to exhibit these data, but is not obliged by this standard to provide copies for retention.

12.3 Classification of Medical Devices

The standard addresses several groups of medical devices. The groups are as follows:

- general medical device
- active medical device
- active implantable medical device
- implantable medical device
- sterile medical device.

The general medical device is defined as any instrument, apparatus, appliance, material, or other article, whether used alone or in combination, including the software necessary for its proper application, intended by the manufacturer for human use for the purpose of:

- diagnosis, prevention, monitoring, treatment, or alleviation of disease
- diagnosis, monitoring, treatment, or alleviation of or compensation for an injury or handicap
- investigation, replacement, or modification of the anatomy or of a physiological process
- control of conception

and which does not achieve its principal intended action in or on the human body by pharmacological, immunological, or metabolic means, but which may be assisted in its function by such means.

An active medical device is defined as any medical device relying for its functioning on a source of electrical energy or any source of power other than that directly generated by the human body or gravity.

An active implantable medical device is any active medical device which is intended to be totally or partially introduced, surgically or medically, into the human body or by medical intervention into a natural orifice, and which is intended to remain after the procedure.

An implantable medical device is any medical device intended:

- to be totally or partially introduced into the human body or a natural orifice, or
- to replace an epithelial surface or the surface of the eye,

by surgical intervention, which is intended to remain after the procedure for at least 30 days and which can only be removed by medical or surgical intervention.

A sterile medical device is any medical device labeled *Sterile.*

12.4 General Provisions

The standard follows the format of ISO 9001:1994, listing the twenty clauses and adding requirements specifically for medical devices. Where no additional requirements for medical devices are necessary, the requirement states that the requirements of ISO 9001 shall apply.

12.5 Guidance Document

To assist in the understanding of the requirements of ISO 13485, an international guidance document has been prepared. The document provides general guidance on the implementation of quality systems for medical devices based on ISO 13485. Such quality systems include those of the European Union Medical Device Directives and the Good Manufacturing Practice requirements currently in preparation in Canada, Japan, and the United States. The document may be used for systems based on ISO 13488 by the omission of sub-clause 4.4.

The guidance document describes concepts and methods to be considered by medical device manufacturers who are establishing and maintaining quality systems. The document describes examples of ways in which the quality system requirements can be met. It is also recognized that there may be alternative methods that are better suited to a particular device or manufacturer. The guidance document is not intended to be directly used for assessment of quality systems.

References

ISO/TC/210/WG1, *Draft of ISO/DIS 13485: Quality systems - Medical devices - Supplementary requirements to ISO 9001*. Arlington: Association for the Advancement of Medical Instrumentation (Secretariat), 1995.

International Organization for Standardization, *First Draft of Quality Systems - Medical Devices - Guidance on the Application of ISO 13485 and ISO 13488.* Arlington: Association for the Advancement of Medical Instrumentation (Secretariat), 1995.

Chapter 13

ISO 13485 Requirements

The standard specifies, in conjunction with ISO 9001, the quality system requirements for the design development, production, and where relevant, installation and servicing of medical devices. This standard, in conjunction with ISO 9001 is applicable where there is a need to assess a medical device manufacturer's quality system or when a regulatory requirement specifies that this standard will be used for such assessment.

13.1 Management Responsibility

13.1.1 Requirements

All requirements of ISO 9001 apply.

13.1.2 Compliance

Compliance is as discussed in Section 7.1.2.

13.2 Quality System

13.2.1 Requirements

All requirements of ISO 9001 apply. The following is a particular requirement for medical devices:

Clause 4.2.1 The manufacturer must establish and document the specified requirements.

Clause 4.2.3 The manufacturer must establish and maintain a file containing documents defining the product specifications, including complete manufacturing and quality assurance specifications for each type/model of medical.

13.2.2 Compliance

The manufacturer must develop and maintain a document which contains the specified requirements for a particular product. The requirements must be developed from customer and market input. The requirements document should be placed under revision control in order to track changes.

A project file or design history file must be developed for each device. The file must contain all the appropriate documents that define the requirements of the device, detail the design and development of the device, and the manufacturing and quality assurance specifications. The file may be hard copy or electronic in nature. When both exist, references to documents in the hard copy file should be made in the electronic file and vice versa. The file must be controlled. An index for the file is helpful in determining the location of specific documents within the file.

13.3 Contract Review

13.3.1 Requirements

All requirements of ISO 9001 apply.

13.3.2 Compliance

Compliance is as discussed in Section 7.3.2.

13.4 Design Control

13.4.1 Requirements

All requirements of ISO 9001 apply. The following is a particular requirement for medical devices:

<u>Clause 4.4.7</u>	If appropriate, the manufacturer must document and maintain records of clinical investigations and risk analysis as part of the design verification activities.
<u>Clause 4.4.8</u>	If appropriate, the supplier must document and maintain records of clinical investigation and risk analysis as part of the design validation activities.

13.4.2 Compliance

Design verification ensures design output meets design input. It commonly consists of design reviews supported by qualification tests and demonstrations, alternative calculations, and design comparisons. Clinical evaluation and risk analysis may be involved in the verification of the design. The conduct of clinical investigations should conform to applicable regulations and standards.

Design validation goes beyond the purely technical issues of verifying that the design output meets the design input, and is intended to ensure that the product meets user requirements. This may involve consideration of who the user really is, the operating instructions, and any restriction on the use of the product. Clinical evaluation and risk analysis may be involved in the verification of the design. The conduct of clinical investigations should conform to applicable regulations and standards.

13.5 Document and Data Control

13.5.1 Requirements

All requirements of ISO 9001 apply. The following is a particular requirement for medical devices:

Clause 4.5.2 — The manufacturer must define the period for which at least one copy of obsolete documents will be retained. This period must ensure that specifications to which medical devices have been manufactured are available for at least the lifetime of the medical device, as defined by the manufacturer.

13.5.2 Compliance

The manufacturer's system should provide a clear and precise control of procedures and responsibilities for approval, issue, distribution, and administration of documentation, including the removal and possibly preservation of obsolete documents. This can be accomplished, for example, by maintaining a master list of documents identifying level of approval, distribution, and revision status.

The manufacturer must keep the appropriate design documentation for each revision of a device for a specified period of time. This time period must be, at a minimum, the time the particular revision may exist in the field and be subject to maintenance by representatives of the manufacturer or a third party service organization. This time period must be defined and listed in a document specifically addressing maintenance of obsolete documents.

13.6 Purchasing

13.6.1 Requirements

All requirements of ISO 9001 apply. The following is a particular requirement for medical devices:

Clause 4.6.3 To the extent required by the particular requirements for traceability in clause 4.8, the manufacturer must retain copies of relevant purchasing documents.

13.6.2 Compliance

Successful procurement of supplies begins with a clear definition of the purchasing requirement. Formal procedures should allow the manufacturer of a medical device to identify the requirements and relevant information necessary to ensure that nothing purchased causes the product to fail to conform to its specification.

Purchasing documents must be maintained for a period of time specified in a document addressing maintenance of design documentation. This time period should, at a minimum, be as long as a device containing the particular purchased component or assembly is active in the field and potentially subject to regulatory or legal activity.

13.7 Control of Customer-Supplied Product

13.7.1 Requirements

All requirements of ISO 9001 apply.

13.7.2 Compliance

Compliance is as discussed in Section 7.7..

13.8 Product Identification and Traceability

13.8.1 Requirements

All requirements of ISO 9001 apply. The following is a particular requirement for medical devices:

<u>Clause 4.8</u> The manufacturer must establish and maintain procedures to ensure that medical devices received for refurbishing are identified and distinguished at all times from normal production.

The manufacturer must establish, document, and maintain procedures for traceability. The procedures shall define the extent of traceability and facilitate corrective action.

The extent of traceability must include all components and materials used and records of the environmental conditions.

13.8.2 Compliance

The manufacturer must develop and maintain documentation that describes the process of refurbishing medical devices. The documents must include the requirement to keep all refurbished devices physically separate from regularly manufactured devices, to avoid the possibility of shipping a refurbished device as new.

The manufacturer must develop and maintain documentation that describes the process of traceability for its medical devices. The documentation shall address the level of assembly within the device that will be traceable. It must also detail a corrective action plan for any nonconformity within that level.

For manufacturers of active implantable and implantable medical devices, the traceability documentation must address all components and materials used within the device and the environmental conditions in which the device was manufactured when these conditions could potentially cause the device not to meet its specified requirements.

13.9 Process Control

13.9.1 Requirements

All requirements of ISO 9001 apply. The following is a particular requirement for medical devices:

Clause 4.9

The manufacturer must establish, document, and maintain requirements for health, cleanliness, and clothing of personnel if contact between such personnel and product or environment could adversely affect the quality of product.

The manufacturer must ensure that all personnel who are required to work temporarily under special environmental conditions are appropriately trained or supervised by a trained person.

For medical devices:

- that are supplied sterile
- that are supplied non-sterile and intended for sterilization before use
- where the microbiological and/or particulate cleanliness or other environmental conditions are of significance in their use
- where the environmental conditions are of significance in their manufacture

the manufacture must establish and document requirements for the environment to which product is exposed.

The manufacturer must establish, document, and maintain requirements for cleanliness of product if:

- the product is cleaned by the manufacturer prior to sterilization and/or its use
- the product is supplied non-sterile to be subjected to a cleaning process prior to sterilization and/or its use
- the product is supplied to be used non-sterile and its cleanliness is of significance in use, or
- process agents are to be removed from the product during manufacture.

If appropriate, the product cleaned in accordance with the first or second bullet point above need not be subject to the preceding particular requirements prior to the cleaning procedure.

The manufacturer must establish and document requirements for maintenance activities when such activities may affect product quality. Records of such maintenance must be kept.

If appropriate, the manufacturer must establish and document both instructions and acceptance criteria for installing and checking the medical device. Records of installation and checking performed by the manufacturer or his authorized representative must be retained. If the contract allows installation other than by the manufacturer or their authorized representative, the manufacturer must provide the purchaser with written instructions for installation and checking.

The manufacturer must ensure that the quality records relating to processes which cannot be fully verified by subsequent inspection and testing of the product, must identify:

- the work instruction used
- the date the special process was performed
- the identity of the operator of the special process.

For sterile medical devices, the manufacturer must subject the medical devices to a validated sterilization process and record all the control parameters of the sterilization process.

The supplier must verify commercially obtained computer software and validate customized computer software for its intended use according to established and maintained documented procedure when computerized systems are used as part of the manufacturer's quality system. The results of verification and validation must be recorded.

13.9.2 Compliance

The manufacturer must establish and maintain documentation detailing requirements for health, cleanliness, and personal clothing to be used during manufacturing, where contact between such personnel and the product and/or environment could adversely affect the quality of the product. These procedures are especially important with regard to such areas as clean rooms and areas sensitive to electrostatic discharge.

All personnel working under special environmental conditions or performing special processes and/or functions must be properly trained to successfully operate under those conditions, or be supervised by an individual who has been trained. The training for these individuals must be included in the individual's training record, including details of the training, date of training, and signature of the trainer.

The manufacturer must establish and maintain documentation specifying the requirements for the environment to which medical devices that are supplied sterile, supplied non-sterile and intended for sterilization before use, where microbiological and/or particulate cleanliness are of significance, and where the environmental conditions are of significance during manufacture are exposed. Such procedures must include details of the methods of control of the environment and how it is to be monitored.

Procedures must be established and maintained that detail cleanliness requirements for products which are cleaned by the manufacturer prior to sterilization and/or its use, supplied non-sterile and subjected to a cleaning process prior to sterilization, supplied to be used non-sterile and its cleanliness is of significance, and where process agents are to be removed from the product during manufacture.

Procedures must be established and maintained which detail maintenance activities, where such activities affect product quality. The procedures must include a requirement for establishing and maintaining records of such maintenance, including product name, type of maintenance performed, date of maintenance, and individual performing the work.

The manufacturer must establish and maintain detailed instructions for installing and checking each medical device. Such instructions must include or reference the acceptance criteria for the device. A record of the installation and check out must be developed and maintained. Such record should include the device name, name of the customer, date of the installation, record of the installation instructions, any problems found during installation, and the name of the individual performing the installation.

Prior to sterilizing medical devices, the manufacturer must have validated the sterilization process and recorded the control parameters and the results of the process, including date and personnel performing the validation.

When computerized systems are used as part of the quality system, the manufacturer must verify commercially obtained computer software and validate customized computer software for its intended application according to established and maintained documented procedures. The results of verification and validation must be recorded.

13.10 Inspection and Testing

13.10.1 Requirements

All requirements of ISO 9001 apply. The following is a particular requirement for medical devices:

<u>Clause 4.10.5</u> For active implantable and implantable medical devices, the manufacturer must record the identity of personnel performing any inspection or testing.

13.10.2 Compliance

For active implantable and implantable devices, personnel performing inspection and testing must be identified. This could be accomplished directly on the inspection or test documentation by use of initials, employee number, or signature.

13.11 Control of Inspection, Measuring, and Test Equipment

13.11.1 Requirements

All requirements of ISO 9001 apply.

13.11.2 Compliance

Compliance is as discussed in Section 7.11.2.

13.12 Inspection and Test Status

13.12.1 Requirements

All requirements of ISO 9001 apply.

13.12.2 Compliance

Compliance is as discussed in Section 7.12.2.

13.13 Control of Nonconforming Product

13.13.1 Requirements

All requirements of ISO 9001 apply. The following is a particular requirement for medical devices:

Clause 4.13.2 The manufacturer must ensure that nonconforming product is accepted by concession only if regulatory requirements are met. The identity of the person authorizing the concession must be recorded.

If the product needs to be reworked, the manufacturer must document the rework in a work instruction that has undergone the same authorization and approval procedure as the original work instruction. Prior to authorization and approval, a determination of any adverse effect of the rework upon product must be made and documented.

13.13.2 Compliance

When concessions are developed for nonconforming product, the concession must be reviewed and approved by appropriate personnel, including the individual responsible for regulatory requirements. The concession should contain the signatures of those individuals reviewing and approving the concession.

Devices that need to be reworked must be reworked according to detailed documentation. The rework documentation must be reviewed and approved according to the same procedures used for the original work instructions. The review must include a review of any adverse effects the rework may have on the product. The results of this review must be documented and maintained.

13.14 Corrective and Preventive Action

13.14.1 Requirements

All requirements of ISO 9001 apply. The following is a particular requirement for medical devices:

Clause 4.14.1 The manufacturer must establish and maintain a documented feedback system to provide early warning of quality problems and for input into the corrective action system.

If this standard is used for compliance with regulatory requirements that require the manufacturer to gain experience from the post production phase, the review of this experience must form part of the feedback system.

All feedback information, including reported customer complaints and returned product, must be documented, investigated, interpreted, collated, and communicated in accordance with defined procedures by a designated person.

If any customer complaint is not followed by corrective action, the rationale must be recorded.

The manufacturer must maintain records of all complaint investigations. When the investigation determines that the activities at remote premises played a part in the complaint, a copy of the report must be sent to those premises.

If this standard is used for compliance with regulatory requirements, the manufacturer must establish, document, and maintain procedures to notify the regulatory authority of those incidents which meet the reporting criteria.

The manufacturer must establish, document, and maintain procedures for the issue of advisory notices and the recall of medical devices. These procedures must be capable of being implemented at any time.

13.14.2 Compliance

The manufacturer must establish and maintain procedures for capturing information from manufacturing and the field and providing feedback to appropriate personnel for corrective action. The procedures must detail the method of information capture, processing of the information, and feedback to appropriate personnel.

All complaints must be investigated and the appropriate corrective action taken to address the problem. Where the activities at a remote site where an important part of the complaint, the site should be sent a copy of the report. Where a customer complaint is not followed by corrective action, the rationale for that action must be documented and maintained.

Procedures must be established and maintained detailing the notification of appropriate regulatory bodies when the complaint may require regulatory activity or intervention.

13.15 Handling, Storage, Packaging, Preservation, and Delivery

13.15.1 Requirements

All requirements of ISO 9001 apply. The following is a particular requirement for medical devices:

Clause 4.15.1 The manufacturer must establish and maintain documented procedures for the control of product with a limited shelf life or requiring special storage conditions. Such special storage conditions must be controlled and recorded.

If appropriate, special provisions must be established, documented, and maintained for the handling of used product in order to prevent contamination of other product, the manufacturing environment, or personnel.

Clause 4.15.4 The manufacturer must establish and maintain documented procedures for the maintenance of labeling integrity and the prevention of labeling mix-ups.

For sterile medical devices, the manufacturer must establish and maintain procedures to ensure that:

- the medical device is represented in a container which maintains the sterility of the medical device, except for those medical devices for which only the inner surfaces of the device are sterile and the device is such that the sterility of the inner surfaces is maintained
- the medical device is capable of being presented in an aseptic manner, if its use so requires

- the package or medical if only the inner surface is sterile, clearly reveals that it has been opened.

For active implantable and implantable medical devices, the manufacturer must record the identity of persons who perform the final labeling operation.

Clause 4.15.6 The manufacturer must ensure that any authorized representative maintains records of distribution of medical devices and that such records are available for inspection.

For active implantable and implantable medical devices, the manufacturer must ensure that the name and address of the shipping package consignee is included in the quality records.

13.15.2 Compliance

Procedures must be established and maintained detailing procedures for the control of product with a limited shelf life or requiring special storage conditions. When addressing product with limited shelf life, the procedures should indicate the method of product use, such as first in, first out (FIFO).

Procedures must be established and maintained detailing special provisions for the handling or used product in order to prevent contamination of personnel, the environment, or other product. The procedure should detail how the product is to be prepared for analysis, without destroying the reason for its return.

Procedures must be established and maintained that detail the packaging and labelling of sterile medical devices. For active implantable and implantable devices, the procedure must require the identification of the individual (s) performing the final labelling operation.

For active implantable and implantable medical devices, the manufacturer must record and maintain the name and address of the shipping package consignee. These must be included in the quality records.

13.16 Control of Quality Records

13.16.1 Requirements

All requirements of ISO 9001 apply. The following is a particular requirement for medical devices:

Clause 4.16 The manufacturer must retain the quality records for a period of time at least equivalent to the lifetime of the medical device defined by the manufacturer, but not less than two years from the date of dispatch from the manufacturer.

The manufacturer must establish and maintain a record for each batch of medical devices that provides traceability to the extent required by clause 4.8 and identifies the quantity manufactured and quantity released for distribution. The batch record must be verified and authorized.

13.16.2 Compliance

The manufacture must develop a procedure which documents the length of time quality are to be retained and maintained. The minimum length of time for retention of the quality records must exceed two years from the date of shipment of the device.

The manufacturer must establish and maintain a record of each batch of medical devices produced. The documentation must contain traceability according to established procedures. It must also identify the quantity of devices manufactured and the quantity released for distribution. The batch record must be reviewed and signed.

13.17 Internal Quality Audits

13.17.1 Requirements

All requirements of ISO 9001 apply.

13.17.2 Compliance

The discussion is as in Section 7.17.2

13.18 Training

13.18.1 Requirements

All requirements of ISO 9001 apply.

13.18.2 Compliance

The discussion is as in Section 7.18.2

13.19 Service

13.19.1 Requirements

All requirements of ISO 9001 apply.

13.19.2 Compliance

The discussion is as in Section 7.19.2

13.20 Statistical Techniques

13.20.1 Requirements

All requirements of ISO 9001 apply.

13.20.2 Compliance

The discussion is as in Section 7.20.2

References

International Organization for Standardization, *Committee Draft 13485: Quality management and corresponding general aspects for medical devices.* 1995.

International Organization for Standardization, *First Draft of Quality Systems - Medical Devices - Guidance on the Application of ISO 13485 and ISO 13488.* Arlington: Association for the Advancement of Medical Instrumentation (Secretariat), 1995.

Chapter 14

IEC 601-1-4

Computers are increasingly used in medical electrical equipment, often in critical safety roles. The use of computing technologies in or as medical devices introduces a level of complexity which is exceeded only by the biological systems of the patients the medical device is intended to diagnose and/or treat. This complexity means that systematic failures can escape practical accepted limits of testing. Accordingly, IEC 601-1-4 goes beyond traditional testing and assessment of the finished medical electrical equipment and includes requirements for the processes by which the medical device is developed, since testing of the finished product is not, by itself, adequate to address the safety of complex medical devices.

This standard is a collateral standard to the general standard IEC 601-1. It requires that a process be followed and that a record of that process be produced to support the safety of medical devices incorporating software-controlled subsystems. The concepts of risk management and a development life cycle are the basis of this standard.

14.1 Scope

IEC 601-1-4 applies to the safety of medical electrical equipment and medical electrical systems incorporating programmable electronic subsystems. It specifies requirements for the process by which a programmable electronic subsystem is designed. This standard also serves as the basis of requirements of particular standards, including serving as a guide to safety requirements for the purpose of reducing and managing risk. The standard covers:

- the requirement specification
- architecture
- detailed design and implementation including software development
- modification
- verification and validation
- marking and accompanying documents.

14.2 General Provisions

OEC 601-1-4 requires that a process with certain elements be established and followed because the subject technology is not amenable to pass/fail tests on the finished product. The approach is to state what is required, leaving the user to determine how this is achieved. This is similar to the approach taken in the ISO 9000 series. As users are expected to be qualified, detail has been kept to the a minimum. Iteration of the process is expected, but no requirements have been given because the need to repeat processes is unique to a particular project. Iterations also arise from the more detailed understanding that emerges during the design process.

As part of the process, documentation is required because it is necessary for process control. In addition, inspection of the documentation permits checking compliance with the process requirements of this standard. A risk management summary is part of the documentation to ensure that safety issues and measures can be readily comprehended during and at the end of the process.

While not unique to programmable electronic systems, risk management is emphasized in order to address the essential complexity of the subject technology and to ensure the early identification of hazards. If subsequent rigor is to be effective in addressing safety, such early identification of hazards is necessary. The requirements are intended to be a framework within which experience, insight, and judgement are applied to manage risk successfully. The level of detail has been chosen to be appropriate to this standard. A risk management summary is required to ensure the risks of identified hazards are controlled.

Software and other systematic failures do not fit into the concept of likelihood or probability as events in themselves. A major objective of this standard, however, is to reduce the likelihood of systematic errors present. Another related concern is the likelihood of the hazardous error being encountered in use. While seldom quantifiable, these components of the risk associated with systematic errors are carefully considered in any responsible design process. Risk estimation is a necessary step both in determining where to focus design effort and in judging results.

14.3 Risk

The term risk is defined as the probable rate of occurrence of a hazard causing harm and the degree of severity of the harm. The concept has two elements: 1) the possibility of a hazardous event and 2) the severity of the consequence of that hazardous event.

The probability of occurrence may be classified into various levels as described in Table 14-1. The levels of severity may be classified as indicated in Table 14-2. The US Food and Drug Administration has rated medical devices into three levels of concern, major, moderate, and minor. The severity levels in Table 14-2 approximate the FDA levels as follows:

Major	Critical
Moderate	Marginal
Minor	Negligible

Risk may be graphed into three regions when analyzing the probabilities of occurrence and the levels of severity (Figure 14.1). The risk regions are classified as the intolerable region, the as low as reasonably practical region, and the broadly acceptable region.

The intolerable region contains the risk of some hazards that are so bad, a system which incorporated them would not be tolerated. A risk in this region must be reduced either by reducing the severity and/or the probability of occurrence.

Probability of Occurrence	Consequence
Frequent	Likely to occur often
Probable	Will occur several times in the lifetime of the device
Occasional	Likely to occur sometime in the lifetime of the device
Remote	Unlikely to occur, but possible
Improbable	Probability of occurrence indistinguishable from zero
Impossible	Probability of occurrence is zero

Table 14-1 Probability of Occurrence and Consequences (From Fries, 1997)

The region between the intolerable and the broadly acceptable is called the as low as reasonably practical (ALARP) region. In this region, risks are reduced to the lowest practical level, bearing in mind the benefits of accepting the risk and the cost of further risk reduction. Any risk must be reduced to a level which is as low as reasonably practical. Near the limit of intolerable risk, risks would normally be reduced, even at considerable cost. Risks near the broadly acceptable region would be reduced if reasonable to do so, but the measure of reasonableness will have been raised. If the risk falls between the intolerable and broadly acceptable, and if the ALARP principle has been applied, the resulting risk is the acceptable risk for that particular hazard.

In some cases, either the severity and/or the probability of occurrence is so low that the risk is negligible compared with the risk of other hazards that are accepted. Risk reduction, in this broadly acceptable region, need not be actively pursued.

14.4 Deciding on Acceptable Risk

There is no standard that defines acceptable risk. It is planned that particular device standards will give guidance. Often acceptable risk has to be established on a case by case basis, based on the intended application and the operating environment. Some guidance may be obtained by interpreting the single fault condition and from the performance of similar equipment already in use.

Severity Level	Consequence
Catastrophic	potential of resulting in multiple deaths or serious injuries
Critical	potential of resulting in death or serious injury
Marginal	potential of resulting in injury
Negligible	little or no potential to result in injury

Table 14-2 Severity Levels and Consequences (From Fries, 1997)

In the case of medical equipment, it may be that the risk associated with the equipment would be acceptable if the prognosis was improved. This cannot be used as an excuse for unnecessary risk.

14.5 Factors Important to Medical Device Risk Assessment

The FDA's experience with medical devices suggest that the factors that are important to medical device risk assessment relate to the device itself and to how it is used. Table 14-3 shows those categories and the major elements of each.

14.5.1 Device Design and Manufacture

A device can present a hazard if it is poorly manufactured or if insufficient attention is paid to design elements that influence performance. For example, the failure to design a structural component to resist the stress to which it will be subjected could lead to its fracture. Quality control or quality assurance during manufacturing may not correct the problem. The FDA's experience suggests strongly that good manufacturing practices do not eliminate inherently bad designs, and could simply ensure that a bad design is faithfully produced. Alternatively, inattention to manufacturing quality assurance could unintentionally cause a device defect.

Device hazards can also be considered in terms of whether the product does something that can cause harm, or whether the product fails to provide a benefit that it should. For example, patients and health professionals may be

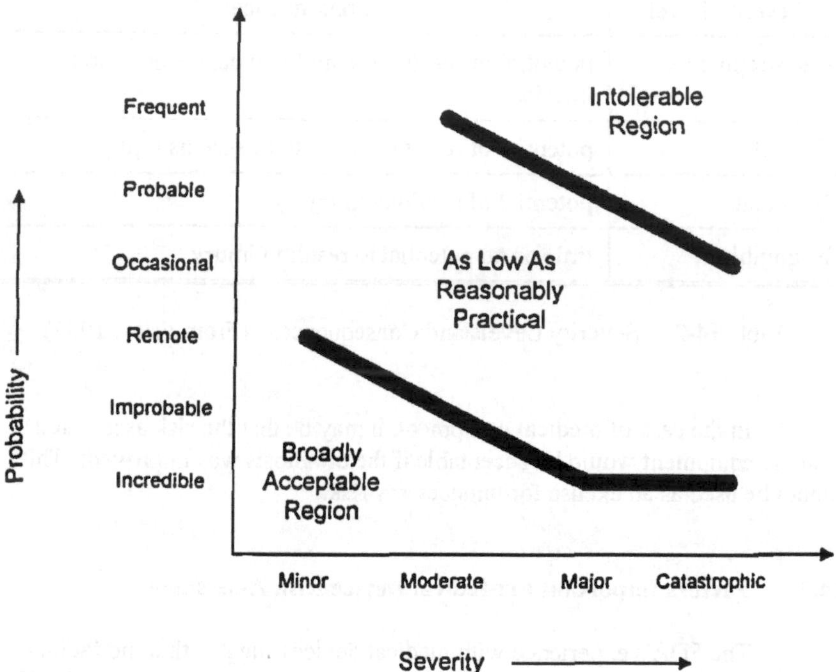

Figure 14-1 Risk probability regions. (From Fries, 1997)

harmed by an electric shock from a supposedly insulated device. A missed diagnosis, on the other hand, could lead to inappropriate therapy or no therapy at all, each with dire consequences for the patient. It is important to the eventual management of risk to determine if the hazard arises from omission or commission.

14.5.2 Materials

Materials from which devices are made are a part of the design and manufacturing process considerations. Proper design includes selection of appropriate materials. Good manufacturing practice includes process validation to ensure that the material's properties are not compromised. It is also important to consider materials separately when the device in question is applied to or implanted in the body. In this regard, both the effect of the material on the body and the effect of the body on the material are important.

For the Device	For Device Use
Design	Adequacy of instructions
Human Factors Engineering	Training of users
Manufacturing of quality control and quality assurance	Interaction with other devices
Materials toxicity	Human Factors Engineering
Materials degradation	

Table 14-3 Major Factors Considered in Medical Device Risk Assessment

14.5.3 Device Users

The FDA's experience has repeatedly and consistently been that how a device is used is a significant part of the overall safety and effectiveness of that device. From the sample collection procedures that can influence the result obtained from an *in vitro* diagnostic device to the poor X-ray film processing techniques that lead to the need for a retake, experience clearly indicates the importance of the user.

The user of a medical device can be a health care professional, a patient, or a family member. There is a large variability in user's skill with devices, due to factors such as education and training, health status, environment, and motivation. Whatever the capability of a particular user, circumstances occur that can be a controlling influence, such as the inattention that can result when a tired individual tries to perform a repetitive task.

The user also represents the decision point on the application of medical technology. The decision may be wrong. Patients may inappropriately rely on over-the-counter devices.

The kinds of hazards that may result from user error are not unusual in themselves. What is unusual is that the incidence of such hazards occurring can range from nonexistent to frequent depending on the influence of the user. Thus, the training of the user and the adequacy of the instructions provided with the device relate directly to assessing the above risks.

14.5.4 Human Factors

Human factors are those device design elements and use conditions that influence how the device and the user interact. This interaction places an additional complexity on the ability to identify the hazards that might be associated with a particular device. Without considering human factors as part of the risk assessment, it would have been difficult to consider the appropriate risk management approach.

14.5.5 Medical Device Systems

The device-intensive nature of certain medical circumstances results in many devices used within close proximity to each other. Such configurations may have been considered by the manufacturer as part of the design, but the ingenuity of device users to devise new systems may outstrip the manufacturer's expectations. Depending on the configuration and number of devices involved, hazards to the patient can result from the interference of one device with another, for example, electromagnetic interference. Users may also attempt to interchange incompatible device components in an attempt at repair and create a risk to the patient. Even if the manufacturer intended for the device to be used in an environment with many others, patients can be at risk because of user behavior in dealing with the total amount of information that must be monitored. Again, developing appropriate problem-solving methods depends on accurate problem identification.

14.6 Risk Management

Risk management is an ongoing process continually iterated throughout the life of a project. Some potential problems never materialize. Others materialize and are addressed. New risks are identified and mitigation strategies are devised as necessary. Some potential problems submerge, only to resurface later. Following the risk management procedures described here can increase the probability that potential problems will be identified, confronted, and overcome before they become crisis situations.

14.7 The Risk Management Process

Many software projects fail to deliver acceptable systems within schedule and budget. Many of these failures might have been avoided had the project team properly assessed and mitigated the risk factors, yet risk management is seldom applied as an explicit project management activity. One reason risk management is not practiced is that very few guidelines are available that offer a practical, step-by-step approach to managing risk.

The risk management process is a multi-step process consisting of:

Identifying the risk factors
Assessing risk probabilities and effects on the project
Developing strategies to mitigate identified risks
Monitoring risk factors
Invoking a contingency plan
Managing the crisis
Recovering from the crisis.

A risk management process should be used throughout the development life cycle. The objective of the process is to manage risk so that it is both less than the maximum tolerable risk and also is as low as reasonably practical. A typical risk management process is shown in Figure 14-2.

14.7.1 Identifying the Risk Factors

A risk is a potential problem. A problem is a risk that has materialized. Exactly when the transformation takes place is somewhat subjective. A schedule delay of one week might not be a cause for concern, but a delay of one month could have serious consequences. The important thing is that all parties who may be affected by a schedule delay agree in advance on the point at which a risk will become a problem. That way, when the risk does become a problem, it is mitigated by the planned corrective actions. In identifying a risk, one must take care to distinguish symptoms from underlying risk factors. A potential delay may in fact be a symptom of difficult technical issues or inadequate resources.

Identifying a situation as a risk or an opportunity depends on the point of view. Is the glass half full or half empty? Situations with high potential for failure often have the potential for high payback as well. Risk management is not the same as risk aversion. Competitive pressures and the demands of modern society require that one take risks to be successful.

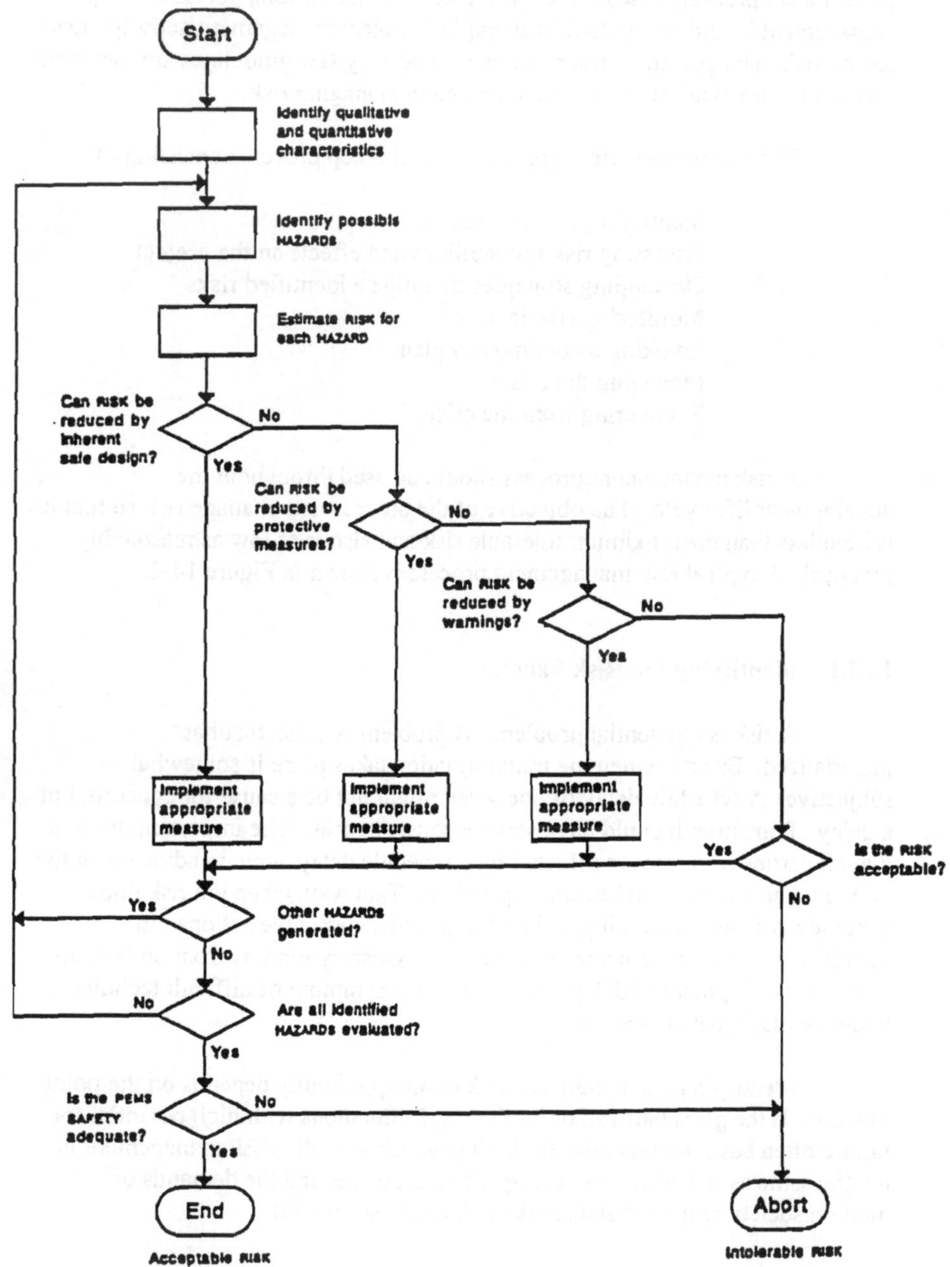

Figure 14-2 Typical risk management process. (From Fries, 1997)

14.7.2 Assessing Risk Probabilities and Effects on the Project

Because risk implies a potential loss, one must estimate two elements of a risk: the probability that the risk will become a problem and the effect the problem would have on the project's desired outcome. For software projects, the desired outcome is an acceptable product delivered on time and within budget. Factors that influence product acceptability include delivered functionality, performance, resource use, safety, reliability, versatility, ease of learning, ease of use, and ease of modification.

Depending on the situation, failure to meet one or more of these criteria within the constraints of schedule and budget can precipitate a crisis for the developer, the customer, and/or the user community. Thus, the primary goal of risk management is to identify and confront risk factors with enough lead time to avoid a crisis.

The best approach is to assess the probability of risk by computing probability distributions for code size and complexity and use them to determine the effect of limited target memory and execution time on overall project effort. Monte Carlo simulation is then used to compute the distribution of estimated project effort as a function of size, complexity, timing, and memory, using regression based modeling. This approach uses estimated effort as the metric to assess the impact of risk factors. Because effort is the primary cost factor for most software projects, one can use it as a measure of overall project cost, especially when using loaded salaries burdened with facilities, computer time, and management, for example.

14.7.3 Developing Strategies to Mitigate Identified Risks

In general, a risk becomes a problem when the value of a quantitative metric crosses a predetermined threshold. For that reason, two essential parts of risk management are setting thresholds, beyond which some corrective action is required, and determining in advance what that corrective action will be. Without such planning, one quickly realizes the truth in the answer to Fred Brooks' rhetorical question, "How does a project get to be a year late?" One day at a time.

Risk mitigation involves two types of strategies: action planning and contingency planning.

Action planning addresses risks that can be mitigated by immediate response. To address the risk of insufficient experience with a new hardware architecture, for example, the action plan could provide for training the development team, hiring experienced personnel, or finding a consultant to work with the project team. Of course, one should not spend more on training or hiring than would be paid back in increased productivity. If you estimate that training and hiring can increase productivity by 10 percent, for example, one should not spend more than 10% of the project's personnel budget in this manner.

Contingency planning, on the other hand, addresses risks that require monitoring for some future response should the need arise. To mitigate the risk of late delivery by a hardware vendor, for example, the contingency plan could provide for monitoring the vendor's progress and developing a software emulator for the target machine.

Of course, the risk of late hardware delivery must justify the added cost of preparing the contingency plan, monitoring the situation, and implementing the plan's actions. If the cost is justified, plan preparation and vendor monitoring might be implemented immediately, but the action to develop an emulator might be postponed until the risk of late delivery became a problem. This brings up the issue of sufficient lead time. When does one start to develop the emulator? The answer lies in analyzing the probability of late delivery. As that probability increases, the urgency of developing the emulator becomes greater.

14.7.4 Monitoring Risk Factors

One must monitor the values of risk metrics, taking care that the metrics data is objective, timely, and accurate. If metrics are based on subjective factors, your project will quickly be reported as 90% complete and remain there for many months. One must avoid situations in which the first 90% of the project takes the first 90% of the schedule, while the remaining 10% of the project takes another 90% of the schedule.

14.7.5 Invoking a Contingency Plan

A contingency plan is invoked when a quantitative risk indicator crosses a predetermined threshold. One may find it difficult to convince the affected parties that a serious problem has developed, especially in the early stages of a project. A typical response is to plan on catching up during the next reporting period, but most projects never catch up without the explicit, planned corrective actions of a contingency plan. One must also specify the duration of each contingency plan to avoid contingent actions of interminable duration. If the team cannot solve the problem within a specified period, typically one or two weeks, they must invoke a crisis-management plan.

14.7.6 Managing the Crisis

Despite a team's best efforts, the contingency plan may fail, in which case the project enters the crisis mode. There must be some plan for seeing a project through this phase, including allocating sufficient resources and specifying a drop-dead date, at which time management must reevaluate the project for more drastic corrective action.

14.7.7 Recovering from the Crisis

After a crisis, certain actions are required, such as rewarding personnel who have worked in burnout mode for an extended period and reevaluating cost and schedule in light of the drain on resources from managing the crisis.

References

Anderson, F. Alan, "Medical Device Risk Assessment," in *The Medical Device Industry - Science, Technology, and Regulation in a Competitive Environment*. New York: Marcel Dekker, Inc., 1990.

Banta, H. David, "The Regulation of Medical Devices," in *Preventive Medicine*. Volume 19, Number 6, November, 1990.

Brooks, F., *The Mythical Man-Month*. Reading, MA: Addison-Wesley Publishers, 1975.

Fairley, Richard, "Risk Management for Software Projects," in *IEEE Software*. Volume 11, Number 3, May, 1994.

Fries, Richard C., *Reliable Design of Medical Devices*. New York: Marcel Dekker Inc., 1997.

IEC, *Draft IEC 601-1-4: Medical Equipment - Part 1: General requirements for safety - 4. Collateral Standard: Programmable electrical medical systems.* Geneva: International Electrotechnical Commission, 1994.

IEC, *Draft First Edition of IEC 601-1-4: Medical Equipment - Part 1: General requirements for safety - 4. Collateral Standard: Programmable electrical medical systems.* Geneva: International Electrotechnical Commission, 1996.

Levenson, Nancy G., *Safeware.* Reading, MA: Addison-Wesley Publishers, 1995.

Levenson, Nancy G., "Software Safety: Why, What and How," *Computing Surveys*. Volume 18, Number 2, June, 1986.

Chapter 15

IEC 601-1-4 Requirements/Compliance

International Standard IEC 601-1-4 was prepared by IEC technical committee 62: Electrical equipment in medical practice. It constitutes a collateral standard to *IEC 601-1: Medical electrical equipment - Part 1: General requirements for safety.* It requires that a process be followed and that a record of that process be produced to support the safety of medical electrical equipment incorporating programmable electronic subsystems. The concepts of risk management and a development life cycle that are the basis of this standard can also be of value in the development of medical electrical equipment that does not include a programmable electronic subsystem.

15.1 Documentation

15.1.1 Requirements

Documents produced from the application of this standard must be maintained and form part of the quality records. These documents must be approved, issued, and changed in accordance with a formal configuration management system.

A risk management summary must be developed throughout the development life cycle as part of the risk management file. The summary must contain:

- identified hazards and their initiating causes
- estimation of risk
- reference to the safety measures including their required safety integrity, used to eliminate or control the risk of hazard
- evaluation of effectiveness of risk control
- reference to verification.

Compliance is checked by inspection of the risk management file.

15.1.2 Compliance

A risk management file is that part of the quality records that includes documents produced from application of this standard. Figure 15-1 contains the contents of the risk management file.

A risk management summary is a document which provides traceability for each hazard and each cause of the hazard to the risk analysis and to the verification that the risk of the hazard is controlled. Figure 15-1 contains the contents of the risk management summary. The risk management summary is required to ensure that the risks of identified hazards are controlled. The summary evolves during the development life cycle and is complete at the completion of the development life cycle.

15.2 Risk Management Plan

15.2.1 Requirements

The manufacturer must prepare a risk management plan. The plan must include:

- scope of the plan, defining the project or product and the development life cycle phases for which the plan is applicable

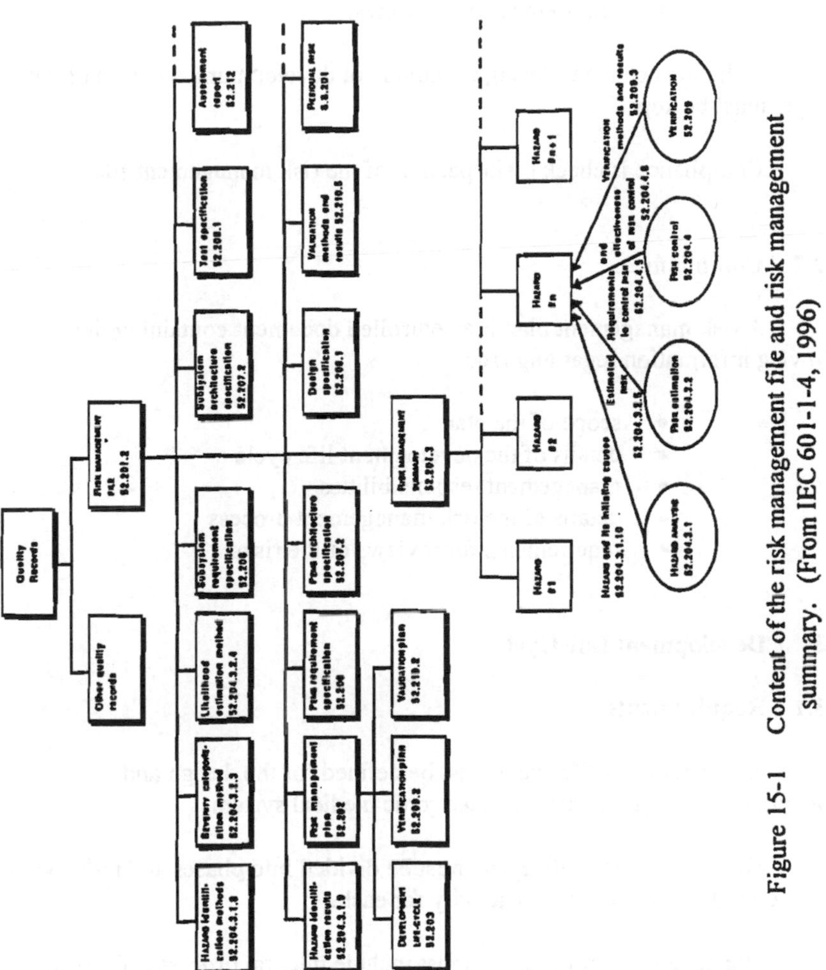

Figure 15-1 Content of the risk management file and risk management summary. (From IEC 601-1-4, 1996)

- the development life cycle to be applied, including a verification plan and a validation plan
- management responsibilities
- risk management process
- requirements for reviews.

If the plan changes during the course of development, a record of the changes must be kept.

Compliance is check by inspection of the risk management file.

15.2.2 Compliance

A risk management plan is a controlled document containing the following information regarding risk:

- scope of the plan
- details of the development life cycle
- management responsibilities
- details of the risk management process
- requirements for reviews of the risks.

15.3 Development Life Cycle

15.3.1 Requirements

A development life cycle must be defined for the design and development of the programmable electronic medical system.

The development life cycle must be divided into phases and tasks, with a well defined input, output, and activity for each.

The development life cycle must include integral processes for risk management and must include documentation requirements.

Risk management activities must apply throughout the development life cycle, as appropriate.

Compliance is checked by inspection of the risk management file.

15.3.2 Compliance

A development life cycle is required to ensure that safety is dealt with in a systematic manner, and in particular, to enable the early identification of hazards in complex systems. The development life cycle must contain phases and tasks with defined inputs, outputs, and activities, including processes for risk management. Documentation requirements are distributed throughout the development life cycle.

15.4 Risk Management Process

15.4.1 Requirements

A risk management process must be used that has the following elements:

- risk analysis
- risk control.

The risk management process must be applied throughout the development life cycle.

Hazard identification must be carried out as defined in the risk management plan.

Hazards must be identified for all reasonably foreseeable circumstances including:

- normal use
- incorrect use.

Hazards considered shall include, as appropriate:

- hazards to patients
- hazards to operators
- hazards to service personnel
- hazards to bystanders
- hazards to the environment.

Reasonably foreseeable sequences of events, which may result in a hazard must be considered.

Initiating causes considered must include, as appropriate:

- human factors
- hardware faults
- software faults
- integration errors
- environmental conditions.

Matters to be considered must include, as appropriate:

- compatibility of system components, including hardware and software
- user interface, including command language, warning and error messages
- accuracy of translation of text in the user interface and instructions for use
- data protection from human intentional or unintentional causes
- risk/benefit criteria
- third party software.

Hazard identification methods appropriate to the development life cycle phase must be used. The methods used must be documented in the risk management file.

The results of the application of the methods must be documented in the risk management file.

Each identified hazard and its initiating causes must be recorded in the risk management summary.

For each identified hazard, the risk must be estimated. The estimation must be based on an estimation of the likelihood of each hazard and/or the severity of the consequences of each hazard.

The severity level categorization method must be recorded in the risk management file.

The likelihood estimation method must be either quantitative or qualitative and must be recorded in the risk management file.

The estimated risk must be recorded against each hazard in the risk management summary.

Risk must be controlled so that the estimated risk of each identified hazard is made acceptable. A risk is acceptable if the risk is less than or equal to the maximum tolerable risk and the risk is made as low as reasonably practicable.

Methods of risk control must reduce the likelihood of the hazard or reduce the severity of the hazard, or both.

Risk control methods must be directed at the cause of the hazard or by introducing protective measures which operate when the cause of the hazard is present, or both, using the following priority:

- inherent safe design
- protective measures including alarms
- adequate user information on the residual risk.

The requirement(s) to control the risk must be documented in the risk management summary.

An evaluation of the effectiveness of the risk controls must be recorded in the risk management summary.

Compliance is checked by inspection of the risk management file.

15.4.2 Compliance

The requirements are intended to be a framework within which experience, insight, and judgement are applied to manage risk successfully. The level of detail has been chosen to be appropriate to this standard. For a particular medical application under consideration, a particular standard may provide more specific methods for managing risk, including pass/fail requirements.

The process is applied throughout the development life cycle so that, as hazard causes are identified, appropriate risk control methods are specified.

15.5 Qualification of Personnel

15.5.1 Requirements

The design and modification of a programmable electronic medical system must be considered as an assigned task in accordance with clause 4.18 of ISO 9001.

Compliance is checked by inspection of the appropriate files.

15.5.2 Compliance

Documented procedures must be established and maintained for identifying training needs. They must provide for the training of all personnel performing activities affecting quality. Personnel performing specific assigned tasks must be qualified on the basis of appropriate education, training, and/or experience, as required. The training process should include:

- evaluation of the education and experience of personnel
- identification of individual training needs
- provision for appropriate training, either in-house or by external bodies
- records of training progress and updates to identify training needs.

Appropriate records of training must be established and maintained.
Training records should include:

- name of the individual
- identification of the training
- purpose of the training
- date the training took place
- location the training took place
- agenda of the training program.

A copy of a certificate of completion should also be placed in the individual's training record.

15.6.1 Requirements

For the programmable electronic medical system and each of its subsystems, there must be a requirement specification. The requirement specification must detail the functions that are risk related, including functions that control risks arising from:

- causes arising from environmental conditions
- causes elsewhere in the programmable electronic medical system
- possible malfunctions.

For each of these functions, the requirement specification must give the level of safety integrity necessary to control the risks.

Compliance is checked by inspection of the risk management file.

15.6.2 Compliance

The requirement specification must detail the functions that are risk related, including functions that control risks arising from:

- causes arising from environmental conditions
- causes elsewhere in the programmable electronic medical system
- possible malfunctions.

Where appropriate, the specification must include requirements for:

- allocation of risk control measures to subsystems and components of the programmable electrical medical system
- redundancy
- diversity
- failure rates and modes of components
- diagnostic coverage
- common cause failures
- systematic failures
- test interval and duration

- maintainability
- protection from human intentional or unintentional causes.

For each of these functions, the requirement specification must give the level of safety integrity necessary to control the risks.

15.7 Architecture

15.7.1 Requirements

An architecture must be specified for the programmable electrical medical system and each of its subsystems. The architecture must satisfy the requirement specification.

Where appropriate, the specification must include requirements for:

- allocation of risk control measures to subsystems and components of the programmable electrical medical system
- redundancy
- diversity
- failure rates and modes of components
- diagnostic coverage
- common cause failures
- systematic failures
- test interval and duration
- maintainability
- protection from human intentional or unintentional causes.

Compliance is checked by inspection of the risk management file.

15.7.2 Compliance

The architecture of the system must meet the requirements of the requirement specification.

15.8 Design and Implementation

15.8.1 Requirements

Where appropriate, the design must be decomposed into subsystems, each having a design and test specification.

Where appropriate, requirements must be specified for:

- software development methods
- electronic hardware
- computer-aided software engineering tools
- sensors
- actuators, human/system interface
- energy sources
- environmental conditions
- programming language
- third party software.

Compliance is checked by inspection of the risk management file.

15.8.2 Compliance

The design must be decomposed into subsystems, each having a design and test specification. Requirements must be specified for:

- software development methods
- electronic hardware
- computer-aided software engineering tools
- sensors
- actuators, human/system interface
- energy sources
- environmental conditions
- programming language
- third party software.

15.9 Verification

15.9.1 Requirements

Verification of the implementation of safety requirements must be carried out.

A verification plan must be produced to show how the safety requirements for each development life cycle phase will be verified.

A reference to the methods and results of the verification must be included in the risk management summary.

Compliance is checked by inspection of the risk management file.

15.9.2 Compliance

A verification plan must be developed and maintained for each medical system. The plan must include:

- scope of the plan
- schedule
- responsibilities
- details of how the safety requirements for each phase of the development life cycle will be verified.

15.10 Validation

15.10.1 Requirements

Validation that safety requirements are met must be carried out. A validation plan must be produced to show that correct safety requirements have been implemented.

The leader of the team carrying out the validation must be independent of the design team.

All professional relationships of the members of the validation team with members of the design team must be documented in the risk management file.

No member of the design team can validate their own design.

A reference to the methods and results of the validation must be included in the risk management file.

Compliance is checked by inspection of the risk management file.

15.10.2 Compliance

A validation plan must be developed and maintained for each medical system. The plan must include:

- scope of the plan
- schedule
- responsibilities
- details of how the safety requirements for each phase of the development life cycle will be validated.

The leader of the team carrying out the validation must be independent of the design team. All professional relationships of the members of the validation team with members of the design team must be documented in the risk management file.

All member of the design team must be independent of the design team.

15.11 Modification

15.11.1 Requirements

If any or all of a design results from a modification of an earlier design, then either all of this standard applies as if it were a new design or the continued validity of any previous design documentation must be assessed under a modification/change procedure.

All relevant documents in the development life cycle must be revised, amended, reviewed, and approved under a document control scheme.

Compliance is checked by inspection of the risk management file.

15.11.2 Compliance

A change to an existing design is treated as a new design with regard to this standard. A change procedure must be established and maintained to ensure all relevant documents in the development life cycle are revised, amended, reviewed, and approved under a document control scheme.

15.12 Assessment

15.12.1 Requirements

Assessment must be carried out to ensure that the programmable electronic medical system has been developed in accordance with the requirements of this standard and recorded in the risk management file. This may be carried out by an internal audit.

Compliance is checked by inspection of the risk management file.

15.12.2 Compliance

An internal audit process must be established to ensure that the medical system has been developed in accordance with the requirements of this standard and pertinent data has been recorded in the risk management file.

References

Fries, Richard C., *Reliable Design of Medical Devices.* New York: Marcel Dekker, Inc., 1997

International Electrotechnical Commission, *Draft of 1st Edition of IEC 601-1-4: Medical electrical equipment - Part 1: General requirements for safety - 4. Collateral Standard: Programmable electrical medical systems.* Geneva: International Electrotechnical Commission, 1996.

International Electrotechnical Commission, *Draft IEC 601-1-4: Medical electrical equipment - Part 1: General requirements for safety - 4. Collateral Standard: Programmable electrical medical systems.* Geneva: International Electrotechnical Commission, 1994.

Chapter 16

ISO 9000-3

ISO 9000-3 provides guidance to organizations that produce software or products that include a software element. The primary rationale for this standard is that software development, supply, and maintenance, unlike other manufacturing processes, does not have a distinct manufacturing phase. The key process is the design phase. The standard offers suggestions regarding appropriate controls and methods that apply to the design phase.

ISO 9000-3 provides guidance for the application of ISO 9001 to software development. Strictly speaking, the ISO 9000-3 guidelines do not establish a so-called sector scheme, not in the sense that there are specific sectors, such as the automotive, aviation, banking, or health care industries. The guidelines exist to bridge the gap between the high level requirements of ISO 9001, which describe the obligations of all quality management systems, and the specifics of applying those principles to software development and use.

It is important to understand the difference between ISO 9001 (the standard) and ISO 9000-3 (the guidelines). Certification and registration of a quality system is to the standard, not to the guidelines. The guidelines offer suggestions or recommendations about things to do or consider that will help a software development organization satisfy the requirements. In most cases, there are other ways to satisfy the standards. One does not have to follow the suggestions made in the guidelines, but should consider what aspects of the standards each addresses. Be sure that those aspects of the standards are being addressed by whatever you do use. Again, it is the standards that must be satisfied, not the guidelines.

16.1 Scope

This international standard sets out guidelines to facilitate the application of ISO 9001 to organizations developing, supplying, and maintaining software. It is intended to provide guidance where a contract between two parties requires the demonstration of a manufacturer's capability to develop, supply, and maintain software products.

The guidelines in this standard are intended to describe the suggested controls and methods for producing software which meets purchaser's requirements. This is done primarily by preventing nonconformity at all stages from development through maintenance.

The guidelines in this standard are applicable in contractual situations for software product when:

- the contract specifically requires design effort and the product requirements are stated principally in performance terms or they need to be established
- confidence in product conformity can be attained by adequate demonstration of certain manufacturer's capabilities in development, supply, and maintenance.

16.2 General Provisions

ISO 9000-3 essentially expands the design stage of the generic ISO 9001 life cycle into a multi-phase software development process, sequenced as follows:

- contract review
- purchaser's requirements specification
- development planning
- quality planning
- design and implementation
- testing and validation

- acceptance
- replication, delivery, and installation
- maintenance.

It also recognizes other software activities that are not dependent on any particular development phase:

- configuration management
- document control
- quality records
- measurement
- rules, practices, and conventions
- tools and techniques
- purchasing
- included software product
- training.

Many paragraphs of ISO 9001 are simply reprinted within ISO 9000-3, presumably to make the guidelines readable as a stand-alone document.

ISO 9000-3 has been structured to suit the information technology community and does not follow the structure of ISO 9001. It provides primary guidance predominantly in the areas of requirements definition, life cycle activities, and configuration management. In other areas, the guidance is minimal and the base standard has in many places been restated for completeness. The guide is essentially divided into three main sections: Quality System – Framework; Quality System - Life Cycle Activities; and Quality System - Supporting Activities.

The framework section consists of management responsibilities, the importance of having a quality plan, and corrective action. The aspects in this section are the purchaser's involvement in the definition of requirements, the nomination of a purchaser representative to act as liaison with the supplier throughout the life cycle of the product, the representative's involvement in the monitoring and review of the requirements, and the progress of the development.

The life cycle activities section contains material that is aimed at those activities which apply to one or more specific parts of the life cycle, regardless of the development model used (e.g., waterfall, spiral, starts V).

The supporting activities section addresses activities that take place after the software is released to the customer. It discusses such actions as configuration management, document control, quality records, measurements, rules, practices, conventions, tools, and techniques.

In judging a quality system, the auditor must recognize the needs of the organization and the complexity of the products. In all cases, ISO 9001 is the source requirement against which noncompliances are referenced. ISO 9000-3 contains the International Standard interpretation of that requirement. Table 16-1 is a mapping of the ISO 9001 clauses and the corresponding ISO 9000-3 clauses.

16.3 Structure of the Standard

ISO 9000-3 is structured and organized based on the premise that associated with each software development project is a life cycle consisting of a set of phases, or defined segments of work. It assumes no particular life cycle, but it does assume the existence of some life cycle with phases.

The standard also presumes that the software product produced is the result of a contractual agreement between a purchaser and a manufacturer, where the manufacturer is the company or organization whose quality system is under review. It emphasizes cooperation and joint efforts between the purchases and the manufacturer. There are clauses in ISO 9000-3 that specifically address the purchaser's responsibility in the contractual agreement.

ISO 9000-3 consists of 22 clauses that do not correspond directly with the 20 clauses of ISO 9001. The 22 clauses are grouped into three major sections:

- Section 4, Quality System - Framework
- Section 5, Quality System - Life-cycle Activities
- Section 6, Quality System - Supporting Activities.

The Framework section deals with activities which are neither phase not project-related, but persist across projects.

The Life-cycle Activities section deals with activities that are related to particular phases of the development process and are project related.

ISO 9001 and ISO 9000-3 Cross Reference		
Quality System Element	ISO 9001 Clause	ISO 9000-3 Clause
Quality System Requirements	4.0	4, 5, 6
Management Responsibility	4.1	4.1
Quality System	4.2	4.2, 5.5
Contract Review	4.3	5.2, 5.3
Design Control	4.4	5.3 - 5.7, 5.10, 6.5
Document and Data Control	4.5	6.2
Purchasing	4.6	6.7
Control of Customer-Supplied Product	4.7	6.8
Product Identification and Traceability	4.8	6.1
Process Control	4.9	5.9
Inspection and Testing	4.10	5.7 - 5.9
Control of Inspection, Measuring, and Test Equipment	4.11	5.7, 6.6
Inspection and Test Status	4.12	6.1
Control of Nonconforming Product	4.13	5.7, 5.9, 5.10, 6.1
Corrective and Preventive Action	4.14	4.4
Handling, Storage, Packaging, Preservation, and Delivery	4.15	5.8, 5.9
Control of Quality Records	4.16	6.3
Internal Quality Audits	4.17	4.3
Training	4.18	6.9
Servicing	4.19	5.10
Statistical Techniques	4.20	6.4

Figure 16-1 Mapping of ISO 9001 versus ISO 9000-3. (From Peach, 1995)

The Supporting Activities section deals with activities that are not related to any particular phase, but apply throughout the process.

16.4 Guidance within the Standard

ISO 9000-3 offers additional guidance for software in the form of:

- clarification of terms peculiar to software and software development
- consideration specifically of software issues
- items to implement.

16.4.1 Considerations

The standard provides the following clarification of terms as they apply to software:

Maintenance

The following are classified as maintenance:

- problem resolution,
- correction of software nonconformities,
- interface modifications,
- software changes to accommodate changes to the hardware,
- functional expansion or performance improvement, and
- software changes to expand or improve an existing function or to improve performance.

Design and Implementation

Design and implementation activities are defined as those which transform the purchaser's requirements specification into a software product.

Configuration Management

Configuration management is described as a mechanism for identifying, controlling, and tracking the versions of each software item. It should:

- uniquely identify the versions of the software items
- identify the versions of each software item that constitute a version of the product

- identify the build status of the software product during development
- control simultaneous updating of a software item
- provide coordination for the updating of multiple products
- identify and track changes to software items.

Purchased Product

Purchased product is described as a software and/or hardware item intended for inclusion in the required end product or a tool intended to assist in the development of the required product.

16.4.2 Considerations

The standard suggests the following list of additional items to consider when designing an ISO 9001 conforming quality system for software development:

Purchaser's Management Responsibility

The purchaser should cooperate with the supplier by providing timely information and prompt response to issues, and by assigning a qualified representative to deal with the supplier of contractual matters.

Joint Reviews

Joint review involving the manufacturer and purchaser should be held to cover software conformance to specifications, verification results, and acceptance test results.

Quality System

The quality system should be an integrated process throughout the entire life cycle ensuring that quality is built into the product as development progresses. Problem prevention should be emphasized. The quality system should be documented in a systematic and orderly manner.

Life Cycle Activities

Development projects should be organized according to a life cycle model.

Contract Review

Contract review should take into consideration:

- identification and assessment of possible contingencies and risks,
- adequate protection of proprietary information,
- the definition of the manufacturer's responsibility with regards to subcontracted work,
- agreed-upon terminology by both parties, and
- the purchaser's capability to meet the contractual obligations.

Purchaser's Requirements Specification

The manufacturer should have a complete, unambiguous set of functional requirements that 1) include all aspects necessary to satisfy the purchaser's needs, 2) are testable, 3) are developed in close cooperation with the purchaser, 4) are subject to document control or configuration management, and 5) specify all product interfaces. The requirements specification should be complete and approved before the development activities start.

Quality Planning

The manufacturer should prepare a quality plan which is updated as the project progresses. Items concerned with each phase should be completely defined when the phase begins. The quality plan should be formally reviewed and approved.

Design

In addition to requirements common to all development phases, consideration should be given to:

- identification of design considerations
- design methodology
- use of past design experience
- subsequent processes, such as testing and maintenance.

Implementation

In addition to requirements common to all development phases, consideration should be given to:

- programming rules
- languages
- naming conventions
- coding rules
- commentary rules
- implementation methodologies.

Reviews

The manufacturer should hold periodic reviews to ensure the requirements are being met and that the plans are being carried out correctly. Design or implementation should not proceed until known deficiencies are resolved or the risk of proceeding is known. Records of reviews should be maintained.

Testing

When testing, consideration should be given to:

- producing a detailed test plan that describes the required testing

- documenting the required hardware and software configuration under test
- recording test results in a meaningful way
- noting discovered problems and their possible impact to any other parts
- notifying responsible personnel of discovered problems
- identifying and retesting areas impacted by any modifications
- evaluating the adequacy and relevancy of tests.

Validation

The complete operation of the product under consideration should be validated under conditions similar to the applications environment prior to making the product available to the purchaser for acceptance testing.

Field Testing

When testing under field conditions, the following should be considered:

- what features need to be tested under field conditions
- the specific responsibilities of the manufacturer and the purchaser for carrying out the test
- restoration of the user environment.

Acceptance

Before carrying out acceptance testing, the manufacturer should assist the purchaser in identifying:

- the time schedule
- the procedures for evaluation
- the software/hardware environments and resources required
- acceptance criteria.

Replication

Replication is the step that is performed before delivery and should consider the following:

- the number of copies to be delivered
- the delivery media
- the required documentation
- copyright and licensing concerns
- custody of master and back-up copies
- the disaster recovery plans
- the length of time the manufacturer is obligated to supply copies.

Installation

For installation, consideration should be given to the roles, responsibilities, and obligations of the manufacturer and purchaser, taking into account:

- schedules
- access to the purchaser's facilities
- availability of skilled personnel
- availability and access to the purchaser's system and equipment
- the need for validation of each installation
- procedures for approval of installation upon completion.

Maintenance

When maintenance is provided by the manufacturer, the following should be considered:

- the preparation of a maintenance plan
- definition, documentation, and agreement on the initial status of the product to be maintained
- the flexibility of a separate support organization
- recording all maintenance information in a predefined format.

Configuration Management

A configuration management system should be used as a mechanism for identifying, controlling, and tracking versions of each software item. A configuration management plan should be developed to describe and plan the configuration management activities.

Product Measurement

Product metrics should be recorded and used to measure and improve the development and delivery process. Some metrics should represent reported field failures and/or defects from the customer's viewpoint. Metrics should be comparable and should be used to report values on a regular basis, identify level of performance, take remedial actions, and establish specific improvement goals.

Included Software

When software other than that produced by the manufacturer is included in the final software product, consideration should be given as to how the included software will be validated for its particular application and how it will be maintained.

16.4.3 Items to be Implemented

The standard suggests the following items to be implemented as part of the quality system:

Quality Plan

A quality plan should be implemented that itemizes the various quality activities that will be undertaken for the project. The quality plan should specify:

- quality objectives in measurable terms
- input and output criteria for each development phase

- identification of the types of tests
- verification and validation activities
- schedules and resources for various test activities
- responsibilities
- the control and correction of defects.

Requirements Specification

The requirements specification should state clearly and unambiguously what is expected from the product that will be produced. In addition to the functional requirements, the specification should consider:

- product performance
- reliability
- safety
- security.

Development Plan

The development plan should contain:

- definition of the project, including objectives
- project organization, including team structure and responsibilities
- development phases
- project management
- development methods and tools
- project schedules
- related plans.

Verification Plan

The standard calls for a verification plan stating how the output from each planned development phase will be verified.

Test Plan

The test plan describes the various levels of test activities planned for the project and should include:

- descriptions of the various test activities
- test case descriptions with test data and expected results
- a statement of required test environments, tools, and software
- specification of the criteria for completion of the various test activities
- personnel requirements and their qualifications.

Maintenance Plan

The maintenance plan specifies all the maintenance activities to be carried out by the manufacturer. It should include:

- definition of the scope of maintenance
- description of the initial status of the product upon delivery
- identification of any required support organizations
- list of maintenance activities
- description of maintenance records and reports.

Release Procedures

Release procedures should specify the procedures for incorporating changes into a software product. These release procedures should specify the ground rules for determining when fixes can be made and when a new release is required. It should also specify the frequency and impact to the purchaser that is allowable for product changes and how the manufacturer will inform the purchaser of changes to the product.

Configuration Management Plan

The configuration plan should specify how configuration management activities will be done and what will be under its control during the project. It should include:

- identification of the organizations involved in and responsible for configuration management

- description of the configuration management activities
- list of configuration management tools, techniques, and methodologies
- specification of when items will be brought under configuration management.

Procedures for Identification of Software Items

The standard calls for procedures for identifying software items during the development process. These procedures should be applied to ensure that the following can be identified for each version of a software item:

- the functional and technical specifications it supports
- the development tools used during its development that affect the functional and technical specifications it supports
- interfaces it provides to other software items and hardware
- documents and computer files related to it.

Procedures for Tracing Software Items

The standard calls for procedures to facilitate traceability of software items. These procedures should allow each version of a software item to be traced back to its origin, including identification of the level of requirements specification supported by the version of the software item.

Procedures for Changing Software Items

The standard calls for procedures to identify, document, review, and authorize any changes to the software items under configuration management. These procedures should include methods to notify those concerned with, or impacted by, the changes.

Status Report Procedures

The standard calls for procedures to record, manage, and report on the status of software items. These procedures should include the status of change requests and the status of approved changes.

16.5 TickIT

Recognition that the process for software development and maintenance is different from that of most other types of industrial products has led to industry pressure to devise an ISO 9000 registration scheme for software. A registration scheme, called TickIT, has been formulated by information technology professionals, led by the TickIT project office of the United Kingdom Department of Trade and Industry and supported by the British Computer Society. The objectives of TickIT are:

- to ensure that the ISO 9000 series of standards is applied appropriately to software
- to ensure consistency of certification within the information technology industry
- to enable mutual recognition of registration across the information technology industry
- to stimulate developers to think about what software quality really is and how it may be achieved.

To ensure the ISO 9000 standards are being applied appropriately, the TickIT scheme requires auditors to use the TickIT Guide, which is based on ISO 9000-3. The TickIT Guide tends to suggest more of how to implement an ISO 9000 conforming quality system than do the standards, which state what must be done. TickIT auditors will look at the quality system for the items suggested in ISO 9000-3.

References

International Standard Organization, *Quality Management and Quality Assurance Standards - Part 3: Guidelines for the Application of ISO 9001 to the Development, Supply and Maintenance of Software.* Geneva: International Organization for Standardization, 1991.

Fries, Richard C., *Reliable Design of Medical Devices.* New York: Marcel Dekker, Inc., 1997.

Peach, Robert W., *The ISO 9000 Handbook, 2nd Edition.* Fairfax, Virginia: CEEM Information Services, 1995.

Schmauch, Charles H., *ISO 9000 for Software Developers.* Milwaukee: ASQC Quality Press, 1994.

Chapter 17

ISO 9000-3 Requirements/Compliance

The standard establishes guidelines to facilitate the application of ISO 9001 to organizations developing, supplying, and maintaining software. It is intended to provide guidance where a contract between two parties requires the demonstration of a manufacturer's capability to develop, supply, and maintain software products. The guidelines describe the suggested controls and methods for producing software which meets purchaser's requirements. This is accomplished primarily by preventing nonconformity at all stages, from development through maintenance.

17.1 Management Responsibility

17.1.1 Requirements

Clause 4.1.1.1 Management should define and document its policy and objectives for, and commitment to quality.

The manufacturer should ensure that this policy is understood, implemented, and maintained at all levels in the organization.

Clause 4.1.1.2.1 The responsibility, authority, and the interrelation of all personnel who manage, perform, and verify work affecting quality should be defined, particularly for personnel who need the organizational freedom and authority to:

- initiate action to prevent the occurrence of product nonconformity
- identify and record any product quality problems
- initiate, recommend, or provide solutions through designated channels
- verify the implementation of solutions
- control further processing, delivery, or installation of nonconforming product until the deficiency or unsatisfactory condition has been corrected.

Clause 4.1.1.2.2 The manufacturer should identify in-house verification requirements, provide adequate resources, and assign trained personnel for verification activities.

Verification activities should include inspection, testing, and monitoring of the development, supply, and maintenance processes and/or product.

Design reviews and audits of the quality system, processes, and/or product should be carried out by personnel independent of those having direct responsibility for the work being reviewed.

Clause 4.1.1.2.3 The manufacturer should appoint a management representative who, irrespective of other responsibilities, should have defined authority and responsibility for ensuring that the requirements of ISO 9001 are implemented and maintained.

Clause 4.1.1.3 The quality system adopted to satisfy the requirements of ISO 9001 should be reviewed at appropriate intervals by the manufacturer's management to ensure its continuing suitability and effectiveness.

Records of such reviews should be maintained.

Clause 4.1.2 The purchaser should cooperate with the manufacturer in a timely manner and resolve pending items.

The purchaser should assign a representative with the responsibility for dealing with the supplier on contractual matters. This representative should have the authority commensurate with the need to deal with contractual matters which include:

- defining the purchaser's requirements to the manufacturer
- answering questions from the manufacturer
- approving manufacturer's proposals
- concluding agreements with the manufacturer
- ensuring the purchaser's organization observes the agreements made with the supplier
- defining acceptance criteria and procedures.

Clause 4.1.3 Regular joint reviews involving the manufacturer and purchaser should be scheduled to cover the following aspects as appropriate:

- continued fitness of the software items to meet purchaser needs
- conformance of the software to the agreed purchaser's requirements specification
- verification results
- acceptance test results.

The results of such reviews should be agreed and documented.

17.1.2 Compliance

The Quality Policy is the overall intention and direction of an organization with regard to quality as formally expressed by top management. The quality policy must be:

- easy to understand
- relevant to the organization
- ambitious, yet achievable.

To fulfill the requirement, management must define the quality policy, quality objectives, and quality commitment of the organization. Once defined, the policy, objectives, and commitment must be documented. Management must then ensure everyone in the organization understands, implements, and maintains the quality policy. This can be accomplished by posting a copy of the quality policy in frequently used places within the organization, printing cards with the quality policy that employees can carry with them, or providing training programs where the quality policy is emphasized.

A management representative must be appointed who has authority to implement and maintain the quality system. If the management representative has other functions, there should be no conflict of interest with those functions. The management representative should be trained in the details of ISO 9000 and be prepared to coordinate all activities necessary to develop and maintain the quality management system.

17.2 Quality System

17.2.1 Requirements

Clause 4.2.1 The manufacturer must establish and maintain a documented quality system.

The quality system should be an integrated process throughout the entire life cycle, thus ensuring that quality is being built-in as a development progresses, rather than being discovered at the end of the process.

Problem prevention should be emphasized rather than being dependent on correction after occurrence.

The manufacturer should ensure the effective implementation of the documented quality system.

Clause 4.2.2 All the quality system elements, requirements, and provisions should be clearly documented in a systematic and orderly manner.

Clause 4.2.3 The manufacturer should prepare a quality plan as part of development planning.

17.2.2 Compliance

The quality management system must be documented. Documentation should include preparatory work to develop the quality management system, the details of how the quality management system will be implemented, and how the quality management system will be maintained. The documentation of the quality management system is normally done in the form of the Quality Manual and Quality Plans (see Chapter 7).

17.3 Internal Quality System Audits

17.3.1 Requirements

The manufacturer should carry out a comprehensive system of planned and documented internal quality audits to verify whether quality activities comply with planned arrangements and to determine the effectiveness of the quality system.

Audits should be scheduled on the basis of the status and importance of the activity.

The audits and follow-up actions should be carried out in accordance with documented procedures. The result of the audits should be documented and brought to the attention of the personnel having responsibility in the area audited.

The management personnel responsible for the area should take timely corrective action on the deficiencies found by the audit.

17.3.2 Compliance

Documented procedures must be established and maintained for planning and implementing internal quality audits to verify whether quality activities and related results comply with planned arrangements and to determine the effectiveness of the quality management system.

17.4 Corrective Action

17.4.1 Requirements

The manufacturer should establish, document, and maintain procedures for:

- investigating the cause of nonconforming product and the corrective action needed to prevent recurrence
- analyzing all processes, work operations, concessions, quality records, service reports, and customer complaints to detect and eliminate potential causes of nonconforming product
- initiating preventive actions to deal with problems to a level corresponding to the risks encountered
- applying controls to ensure that corrective actions are taken and that they are effective
- implementing and recording changes in procedures resulting from corrective action.

17.4.2 Compliance

Documented procedures must be established and maintained for implementing corrective and preventive action. Any corrective action taken

to eliminate the causes of actual or potential nonconformities must be, to a degree, appropriate to the magnitude of problems and commensurate with the risks encountered.

The manufacturer must implement and record any changes to the documented procedures resulting from corrective and preventive action.

17.5 Contract Reviews

17.5.1 Requirements

Clause 5.1.1 — **The manufacturer should establish and maintain procedures for contract review and for the coordination of these activities.**

Each contract should be reviewed by the manufacturer to ensure that:

- **the scope of the contract and requirements are defined and documented**
- **possible contingencies or risks are identified**
- **proprietary information is adequately protected**
- **any requirements differing from those in the tender are resolved**
- **the manufacturer has the capability to meet contractual requirements**
- **the manufacturer's responsibility with regard to subcontracted work is defined**
- **the terminology is agreed upon by both parties.**

Clause 5.1.2 — **Among others, the following items are frequently found to be relevant in the contract:**

- **acceptance criteria**
- **handling of the changes in purchaser's requirements during the development**

- handling of problems detected after acceptance including quality related claims and purchaser complaints
- activities carried out by the purchaser, especially the purchaser's role in requirements specifications, installation, and acceptance
- facilities and tools to be provided by the purchaser
- standards and procedures to be used
- replication requirements.

17.5.2 Compliance

Procedures for review of each contract must be established and a process established for maintaining them. Contract review procedures should include:

- a definition of the requirements
- the establishment of a method for resolving differences
- the establishment of a method for ensuring the supplier has the capability to meet contract requirements.

Records of review must be documented and maintained.

Procedures for establishing and maintaining a contract review process must be developed and maintained. The basic elements of the contract review process include:

- ensuring the scope of the contract is clearly defined
- adequately documenting the requirements
- identifying and resolving any variations
- ensuring the capability to fulfill the contract exists
- ensuring the technical skills exist in-house or can be acquired
- verify the work can be done for the price
- ensure the work can be delivered according to requirements

- ensuring any amendments to the contract are effectively handled.

17.6 Purchaser's Requirements Specification

17.6.1 Requirements

Clause 5.2.1 — In order to proceed with software development, the manufacturer should have a complete, unambiguous set of functional requirements.

These requirements should include all aspects necessary to satisfy the purchaser's need. These may include:

- performance
- safety
- reliability
- security
- privacy.

These requirements should be stated precisely enough so as to allow validation during product acceptance.

The Purchaser's Requirements Specification should be subject to documentation control and configuration management as part of the development documentation.

All interfaces between the software product and other software or hardware products should be fully specified either directly or by reference in the Purchaser's Requirements Specification.

Clause 5.2.2 — When the manufacturer develops the Purchaser's Requirements Specification document, attention to the following issues is strongly recommended:

- assignment of persons responsible for establishing the Purchaser's Requirements Specification

- methods for agreeing on requirements and approving changes
- efforts to prevent misunderstandings such as definition of terms and explanations of the background of requirements
- recording and reviewing discussion results on both sides.

17.6.2 Compliance

Procedures must be established and maintained to ensure that purchased product conforms to specified requirements.

17.7 Development Planning

17.7.1 Requirements

Clause 5.3.1 The development plan should cover the following:

- a definition of the project including a statement of its objectives with reference to related purchaser or manufacturer projects
- the organization of the project resources including the team structure, responsibilities, use of subcontractors, and non-human resources to be used
- project phases
- the project schedule identifying the tasks to be performed, the resources and time required for each, and any interrelationships between tasks
- identification of related plans such as the quality plan, the configuration management plan, the integration plan, and the test plan
- the development plan should be updated as development progresses and each phase should be defined before

activities in that phase are started. It should be reviewed and approved before execution.

Clause 5.3.2.1 The development plan should define a disciplined process or methodology for transforming the Purchaser's Requirements Specification into a software product. This may involve segmenting the work into phases and the identification of:

- development phases to be carried out
- required inputs for each phase
- required outputs from each phase
- verification procedures to be carried out at each phase
- analysis of the potential problems associated with the development phases and with the achievement of the specified requirements.

Clause 5.3.2.2 The development plan should define how the project is to be managed, including the identification of:

- the schedule of development, implementation, and associated deliveries
- progress control
- organizational responsibilities, resources, and work assignment
- organizational and technical interfaces between different groups.

Clause 5.3.2.3 The development plan should identify methods for ensuring that all activities are carried out correctly, including:

- rules, practices, and conventions for development
- tools and techniques for development
- configuration management.

<u>Clause 5.3.3</u> Progress reviews should be planned, held, and documented to ensure that outstanding resource issues are resolved and to ensure effective execution of development plans.

<u>Clause 5.3.4</u> The required input for each development phase should be defined and documented. Each requirement should be defined so that its achievement can be verified. Incomplete, ambiguous, or conflicting requirements should be resolved with those responsible for drawing up the requirements.

<u>Clause 5.3.5</u> The required output for each development phase should be defined and documented.

The output from each development phase should be verified and should:

- meet the requirements specified at the start of the development phase
- contain or reference acceptance criteria for forwarding to subsequent phases
- conform to appropriate development practices and conventions whether or not these have been stated in the input information
- identify those characteristics of the product that are crucial to its safe and proper functioning
- conform to applicable regulatory requirements.

<u>Clause 5.3.6</u> The manufacturer should draw up a plan for verification of all development phase outputs at the end of each phase.

Development verification should establish that development phase outputs meet the corresponding input requirements by means of development control measures, such as:

- holding development reviews at appropriate points in the development phase
- comparing a new design with a proven similar design, if available
- undertaking tests and demonstrations.

The verification results and any further actions required to ensure that the specified requirements are met should be recorded and checked when the actions are completed. Only verified development outputs should be submitted to configuration management and accepted for subsequent use.

17.7.2 Compliance

Plans for each design and development activity must be established and maintained. Typical plans include:

- description of the activity
- schedule for completion
- list of responsible personnel
- details on the implementation of the plan.

Design plans should be updated as the design evolves.

Design input requirements, including such items as applicable statutory and regulatory requirements, must be identified, documented, reviewed, and maintained. Incomplete, ambiguous, or conflicting requirements must be resolved with those responsible for imposing the requirements.

Design inputs will take into consideration the results of any contract review activities.

Design outputs must be documented and expressed in terms that can be verified against design input requirements and validated. Design outputs must:

- meet the design input requirements
- contain or make reference to acceptance criteria
- identify those characteristics of the design that are crucial to the safe and effective functioning of the product.

These may include storage, operating, handling, maintenance and disposal requirements.

Design outputs must be reviewed and maintained.

At appropriate stages of the design, design verification must be performed to ensure that the particular design stage meets the design-stage input requirements. Verification activity must be documented, including verification protocol, test unit setup, details of the activity, results, an indication of acceptance or failure, personnel performing the activity, and the date the activity was performed.

Design validation must be performed to ensure that the product conforms to the defined requirements. The validation activity must be documented including validation protocol, requirements being tested, test unit setup, details of the activity, results, an indication of acceptance or failure, personnel performing the activity, and the date the activity was performed.

Verification and validation activities must be assigned to personnel who are qualified to perform the required activities. Qualification can be based upon education, experience, and/or on-the-job training. Qualifications of personnel must be documented and maintained.

17.8 Quality Planning

17.8.1 Requirements

Clause 5.4.1 The manufacturer should prepare and document a quality plan to implement quality activities for each software development on the basis of the quality system, and make it understood and observed by the organizations concerned.

The quality plan should be updated along with the progress of the development and items concerned with each phase should be completely defined when starting that phase.

The quality plan should be formally reviewed and agreed by all organizations concerned in its implementation.

Clause 5.4.2 The quality plan should specify or reference the following items:

- quality objectives expressed in measurable terms whenever possible
- identification of types and test, verification, and validation activities to be carried out on product specifications, plans and test specifications together with the methods and tools to be employed
- defined entry and exit criteria for each development phase
- detailed planning of test verification and validation activities to be carried out, including schedules, resources, and approval authorities
- specific responsibilities for quality activities, such as:
    - inspections, reviews, and tests
    - configuration management and change control
    - defect control and corrective action.

The document which describes the quality plan may be an independent document or be a part of another document, or composed of several documents including the development plan.

17.8.2 Compliance

The manufacturer should prepare and document a quality plan to implement quality activities for each software development on the basis of the quality system, and make it understood and observed by the organizations concerned. The quality plan should be updated along with the progress of the development and items concerned with each phase should be completely defined when starting that phase. The quality plan should be formally reviewed and agreed upon by all organizations concerned in its implementation.

The quality plan should specify or reference the following items:

- quality objectives expressed in measurable terms whenever possible
- identification of types and test, verification, and validation activities to be carried out on product specifications, plans, and test specifications, together with the methods and tools to be employed
- defined entry and exit criteria for each development phase
- detailed planning of test verification and validation activities to be carried out, including schedules, resources, and approval authorities
- specific responsibilities for quality activities, such as:
    - inspections, reviews, and tests
    - configuration management and change control
    - defect control and corrective action.

17.9 Design Control

17.9.1 Requirements

<u>Clause 5.5.1</u> The design and implementation activities are those which transform the Purchaser's Requirements Specification into an executable software product. Because of the complexity of software, it is imperative that these activities be carried out in a disciplined manner, in order to produce a product of suitable quality, rather than depending on the test and validation activities for assurance of quality.

<u>Clause 5.5.2</u> In addition to the requirements common to all the development phases, the following aspects inherent to the design activities should be taken into account:

- in addition to the input and output specifications, aspects such as design rules and internal interface definitions should be examined
- a systematic design methodology appropriate to the type of software product being developed should be used

- utilizing lessons learned from past design experiences, the manufacturer should avoid recurrences of the same or similar problems
- the product should be designed to the extent practical to facilitate testing, maintenance, and use.

Clause 5.5.3 In addition to the requirements common to all development activities, the following aspects should be considered in each implementation activity:

- rules, such as programming rules, programming languages, consistent naming conventions, coding and adequate commentary rules should be specified and observed
- the manufacturer should use appropriate implementation methods and tools to satisfy purchaser requirements.

Clause 5.5.4 The manufacturer should carry out reviews or inspections to ensure that the requirements are met and the above methods are correctly carried out. The design or implementation process should not proceed until all deficiencies are satisfactorily corrected or the risk of proceeding is known and accepted.

17.9.2 Compliance

In addition to the requirements common to all the development phases, the following aspects inherent to the design activities should be taken into account:

- in addition to the input and output specifications, aspects such as design rules and internal interface definitions should be examined

- a systematic design methodology appropriate to the type of software product being developed should be used
- utilizing lessons learned from past design experiences, the manufacturer should avoid recurrences of the same or similar problems
- the product should be designed to the extent practical to facilitate testing, maintenance and use.

The following aspects should be considered in each implementation activity:

- rules, such as programming rules, programming languages, consistent naming conventions, coding and adequate commentary rules should be specified and observed
- the manufacturer should use appropriate implementation methods and tools to satisfy purchaser requirements.

17.10 Testing and Validation

17.10.1 Requirements

<u>Clause 5.6.1</u> Testing may be required at several levels from the individual software module, to the integrated system. There are several different approaches to testing and integration.

In some instances, validation, field testing, and acceptance testing may be one and the same activity.

<u>Clause 5.6.2</u> The manufacturer should establish and review test plans, specifications, and procedures before starting testing activities, including:

- the integration, system test, and acceptance test plans
- test cases, test data, and expected results
- types of tests to be performed
- test environment, tools, and test software

- the criteria on which the completion of the test will be judged
- user documentation
- personnel required and associated training requirements.

Clause 5.6.3 Special attention should be paid to the following aspects of testing:

- the test results should be recorded to the level defined in the relevant specification
- any discovered problems and their possible impacts to any other parts of the software should be noted and those responsible notified so the problem can be tracked until they are solved
- areas impacted by any modifications should be identified and retested
- test adequacy and relevancy should be evaluated
- the hardware and software configuration during testing should be considered.

Clause 5.6.4 Before offering the product for delivery and purchaser acceptance, the manufacturer should validate its operation as a complete product and under conditions similar to the application environment as specified in the contract.

Clause 5.6.5 Where testing under field conditions is required the following concerns should be addressed:

- the features to be tested in the field environment
- the specific responsibilities of the supplier and purchaser for carrying out and evaluating the test
- restoration of the user environment.

17.10.2 Compliance

The manufacturer should establish and review test plans, specifications, and procedures before starting testing activities, including:

- the integration, system test, and acceptance test plans
- test cases, test data, and expected results
- types of tests to be performed
- test environment, tools, and test software
- the criteria on which the completion of the test will be judged
- user documentation
- personnel required and associated training requirements.

Special attention should be paid to the following aspects of testing:

- the test results should be recorded to the level defined in the relevant specification
- any discovered problems and their possible impacts to any other parts of the software should be noted and those responsible notified so the problem can be tracked until solved
- areas impacted by any modifications should be identified and retested
- test adequacy and relevancy should be evaluated
- the hardware and software configuration during test should be considered.

17.11 Acceptance

17.11.1 Requirements

Clause 5.7.1 — When the manufacturer is ready to deliver the validated product, the purchaser should judge whether or not the product is acceptable according to previously agreed criteria and in a manner specified in the contract.

The method of handling problems detected during the acceptance procedure and their disposition should be agreed between the purchaser and manufacturer and documented.

Clause 5.7.2 Before carrying out acceptance activities, the manufacturer should assist the purchaser to identify the following:

- tune schedule
- procedures for evaluation
- software /hardware environments and resources
- acceptance criteria.

Clause 5.7.3.1 Replication is a step which should be conducted prior to delivery. In providing for replication, consideration should be given to the following:

- number of copies of each software item to be delivered
- type of media for each software item including format and version in human residual form
- the stipulation of required documentation
- copyright and licensing concerns addressed and agreed to
- custody of master and backup copies where applicable, including disaster recovery plans
- period of obligation of the manufacturer to supply copies.

Clause 5.7.3.2. The manufacturer should deliver as specified in the contract. Provisions should be made for verifying the correctness and completeness of copies of the software product delivered.

Clause 5.7.3.3 The roles, responsibilities, and obligations of the supplier and purchaser should be clearly established, taking into account the following:

- schedule including off-hours and weekends
- availability of skilled personnel
- access to purchaser's facilities
- availability and access to purchaser's systems and equipment
- the need for validation as part of each installation should be determined contractually
- a formal procedure for approval of each installation upon completion.

17.11.2 Compliance

When the manufacturer is ready to deliver the validated product, the purchaser should judge whether or not the product is acceptable according to previously agreed criteria and in a manner specified in the contract.

The roles, responsibilities, and obligations of the supplier and purchaser should be clearly established, taking into account the following:

- schedule including off-hours and weekends
- availability of skilled personnel
- access to purchaser's facilities
- availability and access to purchaser's systems and equipment
- the need for validation as part of each installation should be determined contractually
- a formal procedure for approval of each installation upon completion.

17.12 Maintenance

17.12.1 Requirements

Clause 5.8.1.1 When maintenance of the software product is required by the purchaser, after initial delivery and installation, this should be stipulated in the contract.

The supplier should establish and maintain procedures for performing maintenance activities and verifying that such activities meet the specified requirements for maintenance.

Clause 5.8.1.2 Maintenance activities for software products are typically classified into the following:

- problem resolution
- interface modification
- functional expansion or performance improvement.

Clause 5.8.1.3 The items to be maintained and the period of time for which they should be maintained should be specified in the contract. Examples include:

- program
- data and their structures
- specifications
- documents for purchaser and/or user
- documents for the manufacturer's use.

Clause 5.8.2 All maintenance activities should be carried out and managed in accordance with a maintenance plan defined and agreed beforehand by the manufacturer and purchaser. The plan should include:

- scope of maintenance
- identification of the initial status of the product
- support organization
- maintenance activities
- maintenance records and reports.

Clause 5.8.3 The initial status of the product to be maintained at the beginning of the maintenance stage should be defined, documented, and agreed to by both manufacturer and purchaser.

Clause 5.8.4 It may be necessary to establish an organization, with representatives from both manufacturer and purchaser, to support maintenance activities.

This organization should be flexible enough to cope with unexpected occurrences of problems.

It may also be necessary to identify facilities and resources to be used for the maintenance activities.

Clause 5.8.5.1 All changes to the software carried out during maintenance should be made in accordance with the same procedures, as far as possible, used for development of the software product.

All such changes should also be documented in accordance with the procedures for document control and configuration management.

Clause 5.8.5.2 Problem resolution involves the detection, analysis, and correction of software faults causing operational problems.

When resolving problems, temporary fixes may be used to minimize down time and permanent modifications carried out later.

Clause 5.8.5.3 Interface modifications may be required when additions or changes are made to the hardware system or components controlled by the software.

Clause 5.8.5.4 Functional expansion or performance improvement of existing functions may be required by the purchaser in the maintenance stage.

Clause 5.8.6 All maintenance activities should be recorded in predefined formats and retained.

Rules for the submission of maintenance reports should be established and agreed upon by the manufacturer and purchaser.

The maintenance records should include the following items for each software item being maintained:

- list of requests for assistance or problem reports that have been received and the current status of each
- organization responsible for responding to requests for assistance or implementing the appropriate corrective actions
- priorities that have been assigned to the corrective actions
- results of the corrective actions
- statistical data on fault occurrences and maintenance activities.

The record of the maintenance activities may be utilized for evaluation and enhancement of the software product and for improvement of the quality system itself.

Clause 5.8.7 The manufacturer and purchaser should agree and document procedures for incorporating changes in a software product resulting from the need to maintain performance. These procedures should include:

- ground rules to determine where localized *patches* may be incorporated or release of a complete updated copy of the software product is necessary
- descriptions of the types of releases depending on their frequency and/or impact on the purchaser's operations and ability to implement changes at any point in time
- methods by which the purchaser will be advised of current or planned future changes
- methods to confirm that changes implemented will not introduce other problems

- requirements for records indicating which changes have been implemented and at what locations for multiple products/sites.

17.12.2 Compliance

When maintenance of the software product is required by the purchaser, after initial delivery and installation, this should be stipulated in the contract. The supplier should establish and maintain procedures for performing maintenance activities and verifying that such activities meet the specified requirements for maintenance.

All maintenance activities should be carried out and managed in accordance with a maintenance plan defined and agreed beforehand by the manufacturer and purchaser. The plan should include:

- scope of maintenance
- identification of the initial status of the product
- support organization
- maintenance activities
- maintenance records and reports.

Problem resolution involves the detection, analysis, and correction of software faults causing operational problems. When resolving problems, temporary fixes may be used to minimize down time and permanent modifications carried out later.

17.13 Configuration Management

17.13.1 Requirements

<u>Clause 6.1.1</u> The configuration management system should:

- uniquely identify the official versions of each software item
- identify the versions of each software item which together constitute a specific version of a complete product

- identify the build status of software products in development or delivered and installed
- control simultaneous updating of a given software item by more than one programmer
- provide coordination for updating of multiple products in one or more locations as required
- identify and track each change request from suggestion through release.

Clause 6.1.2 The manufacturer should develop and implement a configuration management plan, which includes:

- the organizations involved in configuration management and responsibilities assigned to each of them
- configuration management activities to be carried out
- configuration management tools, techniques, and methodologies to be used.

Clause 6.1.3.1 The manufacturer should establish and maintain procedures for identifying software items during all phases starting from specification through development, replication, and delivery.

Where required by contract, these procedures may also apply after delivery of the product.

Each individual software item should have a unique identification.

Procedures should be applied to ensure that the following can be identified for each version of a software item:

- the functional and technical specifications
- all development tools which affect the functional and technical specifications
- all interfaces to other software items and to hardware
- all documents and computer files related to the software item.

The identification of a software item should be handled in such a way that the relationship between the item and the contract requirements can be demonstrated.

For released products, there should be procedures to facilitate traceability of the software item or product.

Clause 6.1.3.2 The manufacturer should establish and maintain procedures to identify, document, review, and authorize any changes to the software items under configurations management.

All changes to software items should be carried out in accordance with these procedures.

Before a change is made official, its validity should be confirmed and the effects on other items should be identified and thoroughly examined.

Methods to notify the changes to those concerned and to show the traceability between changes and modified parts of software items should be provided.

Clause 6.1.3.3 The manufacturer should establish and maintain procedures to record, manage, and report on the status of software items, change requests, and the implementation of approved changes.

17.13.2 Compliance

The manufacturer should develop and implement a configuration management plan, which includes:

- the organizations involved in configuration management and responsibilities assigned to each of them
- configuration management activities to be carried out
- configuration management tools, techniques, and methodologies to be used.

The manufacturer should establish and maintain procedures for identifying software items during all phases starting from specification through development, replication, and delivery. Procedures should be applied to ensure that the following can be identified for each version of a software item:

- the functional and technical specifications
- all development tools which affect the functional and technical specifications
- all interfaces to other software items and to hardware
- all documents and computer files related to the software item.

The manufacturer should establish and maintain procedures to record, manage, and report on the status of software items, change requests, and the implementation of approved changes.

17.14 Document Control

17.14.1 Requirements

Clause 6.2.1 The manufacturer should establish and maintain procedures to control all documents that relate to the contents of ISO 9000-3. This includes:

- the determination of those documents which should be subject to the document control procedures
- the approval and issuing of procedures
- the change procedures including withdrawal and, as appropriate, release.

Clause 6.2.2 The document control procedures should be applied to relevant documents including:

- procedural documents describing the quality system to be applied in the software life cycle
- planning documents describing the planning and progress of all manufacturer activities and the interactions with the purchaser
- product documents describing a particular software product.

Clause 6.2.3 All documents should be reviewed and approved by authorized personnel prior to issue.

Procedures should exist to ensure that:

- the pertinent issues of appropriate documents are available at appropriate locations where operations essential to the effective functioning of the quality system are performed
- obsolete documents are promptly removed from appropriate points of issue or use.

Where use is made of computer files, special attention should be paid to appropriate approval, distribution, and archiving procedures.

Clause 6.2.4 Changes to documents should be reviewed and approved by the same functions/organizations that performed the original review and approval unless specifically designated otherwise.

The designated organizations should have access to pertinent background information upon which to base their review and approval.

Where practical, the nature of the change should be identified in the document or the appropriate attachments.

A master list or equivalent document control procedures should be established to identify the current version of documents in order to preclude the use of non-applicable documents.

Documents should be reissued after a practical number of changes have been made.

17.14.2 Compliance

Procedures must be established and maintained that describe the control of all documents and data. Documents and data can be in the form of any type of media, including hard copy or electronic media. Control must ensure:

- the pertinent issues of appropriate documents are available at all locations where operations essential to the effective functioning of the quality management system are performed
- invalid and/or other obsolete documents are promptly removed from all points of issue or use, or otherwise ensured against unintended use
- any obsolete documents retained for legal and/or knowledge preservation purposes are suitably identified.

Internal written procedures should contain how documentation for these functions should be controlled, who is responsible for document control, what is to be controlled, and where and when is it to be controlled.

Documents and data must be reviewed and approved for adequacy by authorized personnel prior to issue.

17.15 Quality Records

17.15.1 Requirements

The manufacturer should establish and maintain procedures for identification, collection, indexing, filing, storage, maintenance, and disposition of quality records.

Quality records should be maintained to demonstrate achievement of the required quality and the effective operation of the quality system. Pertinent subcontractor quality records should be an element of these data.

All quality records should be legible and identifiable to the product involved.

Quality records should be stored and maintained in such as way that they are readily retrievable in facilities that provide a suitable environment to minimize deterioration or damage and prevent loss.

Retention times of quality records should be established and recorded.

When agreed contractually, quality records should be made available for evaluation by the purchaser or his representative for an agreed period.

17.15.2 Compliance

Documented procedures must be established and maintained for identification, collection, indexing, access, filing, storage, maintenance, and disposition of quality records. Such procedures should ensure records are:

- legible and identifiable to the product involved
- stored/maintained such that they are readily retrievable
- kept in an environment that prevents deterioration or damage.

Quality records must be maintained to demonstrate conformance to specified requirements and the effective operation of the quality management system. Pertinent quality records from vendors must be an element of this data. Records may be in the form of any type of media, such as hard copy or electronic media.

Retention times must be established and recorded. Where required in the contract, quality records must be made available for evaluation by the customer or the customer's representative for an agreed time period. The following should be considered in specifying a minimum time period for retaining quality records:

- the requirements of regulatory authorities
- product liability and other legal issues related to record keeping
- the expected lifetime of the product
- the requirements of the contract.

17.16 Measurement

17.16.1 Requirements

Clause 6.4.1 Some metrics should be used which represent reported field failures or defects from the customer's veiwpoint.

Selected metrics should be described such that results are comparable.

The manufacturer of software products should collect and act on quantitative measures of the quality of these software products. These measures should be used for:

- collection of data and reporting metric values on a regular basis
- identifying the current level of performance of each metric
- taking remedial action if metric levels grow worse or exceed established target levels
- establishing specific improvement goals in terms of the metrics.

Metrics should be reported and used to manage the development and delivery process and should be relevant to the particular software product or application.

Clause 6.4.2 The manufacturer should have quantitative measures of the development and delivery process.

These metrics should reflect:

- how well the development process is being carried out in terms of milestones and in-process quality objectives being met on schedule
- how effective the development process is at reducing the probability that faults are introduced or that any faults introduced remain undetected.

17.16.2 Compliance

Metrics should be used which represent reported field failures or defects from the customer's veiwpoint. Metrics should be reported and used to manage the development and delivery process and should be relevant to the particular software product or application. These metrics should reflect:

- how well the development process is being carried out in terms of milestones and in-process quality objectives being met on schedule
- how effective the development process is at reducing the probability that faults are introduced or that any faults introduced remain undetected.

17.17 Rules, Practices, and Conventions

17.17.1 Requirements

The manufacturer should provide rules, practices, and conventions in order to make the quality system effective.

The manufacturer should review these rules, practices, and conventions and revise them as required.

17.17.2 Compliance

The manufacturer should provide rules, practices, and conventions in order to make the quality system effective. The manufacturer should review these rules, practices, and conventions and revise them as required.

17.18 Tools and Techniques

17.18.1 Requirements

The manufacturer should provide software tools, facilities, and techniques in order to make the quality system effective.

These tools, facilities, and techniques can be effective for management purposes as well as for product development.

The manufacturer should improve these tools and techniques as required.

17.18.2 Compliance

The manufacturer should provide software tools, facilities, and techniques in order to make the quality system effective. These tools, facilities, and techniques can be effective for management purposes as well as for product development. The manufacturer should improve these tools and techniques as required.

17.19 Purchasing

17.19.1 Requirements

<u>Clause 6.7.1</u>	The manufacturer should ensure that purchased product conforms to specified requirements. Purchasing documents should contain data clearly describing the product ordered.

The manufacturer should review and approve purchasing documents for adequacy of specified requirements prior to release.

Clause 6.7.2 The manufacturer should select subcontractors on the basis of their ability to meet subcontract requirements, including quality requirements.

The manufacturer should establish and maintain records of acceptable subcontractors.

The selection of subcontractors and the type and extent of control exercised by the manufacturer will be dependent on the type of product and, where appropriate, on records of the subcontractor's previously demonstrated capability and performance.

The manufacturer should ensure that quality system controls are effective.

Clause 6.7.3 The manufacturer is responsible for the validation of subcontracted work. This may require the manufacturer to conduct design and other reviews in line with the manufacturer's own quality system and if so, such requirements should be included in the subcontract. Any requirements for acceptance testing of the subcontracted work by the manufacturer should be similarly included.

Where specified in the contract, the purchaser or his representative should be afforded the right to determine at source, or upon receipt, that purchased product conforms too specified requirements. Validation by the purchaser may not absolve the manufacturer of the responsibility to provide acceptable product nor may it preclude subsequent rejection.

When the purchaser or his representative elects to carry out validation at the subcontractor's premises, such validation should not be used by the manufacturer as evidence of effective control of quality by the subcontractor.

17.19.2 Compliance

Procedures must be established and maintained to ensure that purchased product conforms to specified requirements.

Vendors must be evaluated and selected on the basis of their ability to meet contract requirements including the quality system and any specific quality assurance requirements. Vendor evaluation should address:

- their ability to meet requirements
- comparison to records of acceptable vendors.

Vendor evaluations must address

- previous performance in supplying similar products
- satisfactory assessment of an appropriate quality system standard by a competent body
- assessment of the vendor by the manufacturer to an appropriate quality system standard
- product compliance with specified requirements
- total cost for the vendor
- delivery arrangements
- periodic review of the performance of the vendor.

The manufacturer must define the type and extent of control it exercises over its vendors. This is dependent upon the type of product, the impact of vended product on the quality of the final product, and, where applicable, on the quality audit reports and/or quality records of the previously demonstrated capability and performance of vendors. Control depends on:

- the type of product
- records of performance.

The manufacturer must also establish and maintain quality records of acceptable vendors.

17.20 Included Software Product

17.20.1 Requirements

The manufacturer may be required to include or use software product supplied by the purchaser or by a third party.

The manufacturer should establish and maintain procedures for validation, storage, protection, and maintenance of such product.

Consideration should be given to the support of such software product in any maintenance agreement related to the product to be delivered.

Purchaser supplied product that is found unsuitable for use should be recorded and reported to the purchaser.

Validation by the manufacturer does not absolve the purchaser of the responsibility to provide acceptable product.

17.20.2 Compliance

The manufacturer may be required to include or use software product supplied by the purchaser or by a third party. The manufacturer should establish and maintain procedures for validation, storage, protection, and maintenance of such product.

17.21 Training

17.21.1 Requirements

The manufacturer should establish and maintain procedures for identifying the training needs and provide for the training of all personnel performing activities affecting quality.

Personnel performing specific assigned tasks should be qualified on the basis of appropriate education, training, and/or experience, as required.

The subjects to be addressed should be determined considering the specific tools, techniques, methodologies, and computer resources to be used in the development and management of the software product. It might also be required to include the training of skills and knowledge of the specific field the software addresses.

Appropriate records of training/experience should be maintained.

17.21.2 Compliance

Documented procedures must be established and maintained for identifying training needs. They must provide for the training of all personnel performing activities affecting quality. Personnel performing specific assigned tasks must be qualified on the basis of appropriate education, training, and/or experience, as required. The training process should include:

- evaluation of the education and experience of personnel
- identification of individual training needs
- provision for appropriate training, either in-house or by external bodies
- records of training progress and updates to identify training needs.

Reference

International Organization for Standardization, *ISO 9000-3: Quality Management and Quality Assurance Standards - Part 3: Guidelines for the application of ISO 9001 to the development, supply, and maintenance of software.* Geneva: ISO, 1990.

Chapter 18

IEC 601-1

IEC 601-1 is an international electrical safety standard recognized in almost all developed countries as a complete set of regulations for the design of electrically safe medical equipment. The standard is published by the Geneva-based International Electrotechnical Committee (IEC). It originated in Europe and was designed to serve as a uniform pan-European standard. Prior to its inception, different countries had different standards, which manufacturers were forced to comply with if they wanted to market their products there. This was very expensive for everyone. More recently, the IEC 601-1 standard has been adopted in most all developed countries, where it may appear under various designations, including UL 2601, EN 60601, or their equivalent. All of these standards are based on the original, but some may incorporate national deviations for a specific country. For example, UL 2601 uses different leakage limits than the original IEC 601-1.

18.1 History

The first edition of IEC 513 was prepared by IEC subcommittee 62A. It was published in 1976 as an IEC report with the title, *Basic Aspects of the Safety Philosophy of ElectricalEequipment Used in Medical Practice.* The preface stated that the report was to be used as a guideline for the standards which were to be issued by IEC technical committee 62.

The report discussed the clinical environment in which medical electrical equipment was used and many of the hazards which were particular to that type of electrical equipment. It identified the need for safety standards in all of the following areas, to ensure the safe use of medical electrical equipment:

- safety standards relating to the design of the equipment
- installation requirements to ensure the safety of electrical equipment in some clinical applications
- user guidelines to ensure that the equipment was maintained and used safely.

The report provided an overall philosophy for developing the IEC 601 series and a rationale for some of the requirements given in the first edition of IEC 601-1.

As a result of applying the philosophy set out in the report, the original approach in IEC technical committee 62 was to divide standards for medical electrical equipment into separate safety and performance requirements. The parent standard and the IEC 601-2-xx series of particular standards were to be restricted to basic safety issues to ensure that during normal use and under certain fault conditions, the equipment would not produce an unreasonable hazard for the patient, the operator, nor the environment. Where required, other performance matters not directly related to physical safety would be set out in a separate series of IEC 601-3-xx performance standards.

The first edition of IEC 601-1 was prepared by IEC subcommittee 62A and published in 1977 with the title, *Safety of Medical Electrical Equipment, Part 1: General requirements.* The scope of the first edition stated that the standard applied to medical electrical equipment intended for use by or under the supervision of qualified personnel in the patient environment, or related to the patient in such a way that the safety of persons or animals in that environment is directly affected. The second edition was prepared by the same committee and published in 1988, and the third edition in 1992.

The standard specified requirements for the transport, storage, installation, use, and maintenance of such equipment under the environmental conditions specified in subclause 1.4 or by the manufacturer or as prescribed in particular standards. Although the standard is primarily concerned with safety, it contains some requirements regarding reliable operation, where this is connected with safety.

IEC 601-1 will be implemented worldwide over the next several years according to the process of global harmonization. Deadlines for implementation are listed in Table 18-1. After these deadlines, equipment must be certified to the IEC 601-1 standard in order to be sold in these locations.

18.2 The Purpose of Safety Testing

The basic purpose of safety testing of medical electrical equipment is to ensure that a device is safe for both the patient and the caregiver. It is particularly important in product development, on the production line, and in the service department. The IEC 6001-1 standard is intended mainly for the first of these areas, but it can also be applied to the other two areas. Safety testing is especially crucial in the design stages because safety must be designed into equipment, not just tested afterwards. By being aware of the standards, designers can plan ahead for safe construction rather than having to troubleshoot problems in a finished product.

However, even when a design has been verified as safe, it will be necessary for the manufacturer to safety-test products at the end of the line, since a safe original design can still be subject to a solder short, miswired connector, or other assembly error that can cause leakage and thus make the product itself unsafe. Only by testing at the end of the production line can the manufacturer be certain it is shipping a safe product to its customers.

18.3 General Provisions

The safety tests contained in the IEC 601-1 standard cover 10 basic areas of concern. They include:

- earth leakage current - essentially the current that flows down through the ground conductor in the line cord back to earth

Country	Applicable Standard	Implementation Date
European Union	EN 60601-1	June 13, 1998
Canada	CAN/CSA-C22.2 No. 601.1-M90	January 1, 2000
United States	UL 2601-1	December 31, 2004

Table 18-1 Implementation Dates for IEC 601-1

- enclosure leakage current - the current that would flow from any accessible enclosure part if a person was to touch it
- applied-part leakage (commonly known as patient lead leakage) - the leakage that flows from or into an applied part or between applied parts
- dielectric withstand - the ability of insulation to withstand high voltage
- ground-bond continuity - the ability of the ground system connections to handle current
- residual voltage - the voltage present in any plug conductor one second after the plug is disconnected from the line
- accessible-parts voltage - the voltage present on any accessible part, including parts covered by service or access doors
- retained energy - the energy stored in any accessible part
- current draw - the current consumed by the product
- power consumption - the power consumed by the product.

During leakage tests, single faults and normal conditions are used to simulate all electrical possibilities that might occur in the field. Single faults essentially represent potential problem conditions. Since it is very unlikely that two or more faults would occur simultaneously, faults are tested one at a time. Typical single faults used in IEC 601-1 include:

- Open safety ground
- Open neutral
- Mains voltage on SIP/SOP
- Mains voltage on applied part
- Insulation shorting
- Open external power-supply ground
- Open external power-supply neutral.

Normal conditions are electrical situations that occur on a daily basis and that are not considered to be a problem. For example, grounding of a patient-applied part would not constitute a fault since this happens every time an ECG lead touches a metal bed frame. Typical normal conditions used in IEC 601-1 include:

- Reversed line
- Functional earth grounded
- Patient lead grounded
- Isolated metal parts grounded
- Reversed mains voltage on SIP/SOP polarity
- Reversed mains voltage on applied-part polarity
- External power-supply functional earth grounded.

Another important aspect of safety testing relates to line voltage and frequency. If you intend to market your product internationally, it is important that it be tested at the worst voltage and frequency, generally 240 VAC at 50 Hz. If, however, you plan to sell it only in the U.S., you can use a voltage/frequency of 120 VAC at 60 Hz. Whichever level you test to, the IEC 601-1 standard requires that you add an additional 10% as a safety margin.

The last critical variable for safety testing is the actual measurement device used. IEC 601-1 calls for the use of a true RMS leakage meter with very specific load. If possible, select a meter with a crest factor of 10 or more and an accuracy of 1% on leakage current. This is what the test labs will use when you bring your product to them for certification. Thus, it is in your best interest to observe the same criteria.

18.4 Classification of Equipment

Equipment is classified according to category, class, and type.

18.4.1 Categories

Equipment is listed in two categories: category AP equipment and category APG equipment. Category AP equipment is defined as equipment or an equipment part complying with specified requirements on construction, marking, and documentation in order to avoid sources of ignition in a flammable anesthetic mixture with air.

Category APG equipment is defined as equipment or an equipment part complying with specified requirements on construction, marking, and documentation in order to avoid sources of ignition in a flammable anesthetic mixture with oxygen or nitrous oxide.

18.4.2 Class

Equipment is listed in two classes: Class I and Class II. Class I equipment is defined as equipment in which protection against electric shock does not rely on basic insulation only, but which includes an additional safety precaution in that means are provided for the connection of the equipment to the protective earth conductor in the fixed wiring of the installation in such a way that accessible metal parts cannot become live in the event of a failure of the basic insulation.

Class II equipment is defined as equipment in which protection against electric shock does not rely on basic insulation only, but in which additional safety precautions, such as double insulation or reinforced insulation are provided, with no provision for protective earthing or reliance upon installation condition.

18.4.3 Type

For purposes of this section, the following definitions apply. An applied part is defined as the entirety of all parts of the equipment, including the patient leads, which come intentionally into contact with patients to be examined or treated. An F-type applied part is defined as an applied part isolated from all other parts of the equipment to such a degree that the patient leakage current allowable in single fault conditions is not exceeded when a voltage equal to 1.1 times the highest rated mains voltage is applied between the applied part and earth.

Equipment is listed in several types: type B equipment, type BF equipment, and type CF equipment. Type B equipment is defined as equipment providing a particular degree of protection against electric shock, particularly regarding allowable leakage current, and reliability of the protective earth connection.

Type BF equipment is defined as Type B equipment with an F-type applied part.

Type CF equipment is defined as equipment providing a degree of protection higher than that for type BF equipment against electric shock, particularly regarding allowable leakage currents and having an F-type applied part.

18.5 Testing

There are ten basic safety testing areas as listed in Section 18.3. Table 18-2 references each test type to the appropriate clause in IEC 601-1.

18.5.1 Earth Leakage Current

Also known as safety-ground current, this is a very critical safety test comprising a sum of all leakages in the product under test. Basically it measures the current flowing back to earth ground through the ground conductor of the line cord. This test needs to be performed under varying normal and single-fault conditions. The standard specifies that this test be made with both opened and closed neutral under all possible combinations of reversed line, grounded functional earth terminal, and grounded patient leads. This makes for 16 different combinations of conditions to test if the equipment has a functional earth and an applied part. If the product under test does not have a functional earth terminal or patient lead, the number of combinations is reduced.

Figure 18-1 provides a schematic for making this test. Note the locations of switches. The switch number references are identical to those used in the standard for easy reference.

All combinations that apply must be tested. If a device does not have one of the settings shown, however, such as Applied Parts, the iterations for that setting may be omitted.

The measured earth-leakage current should not exceed specified limits during any of the steps. The allowable limits are detailed in Table 18-3.

Safety Test Type	IEC 601-1 Clause
Earth leakage current	19
Enclosure leakage current	19
Aplied-part leakage	19
Dielectric withstand	20
Ground-bond continuity	18.f
Residual voltage	15.b, 15.c, 16.a5, 16.c
Accessible-parts voltage	15.b, 15.c, 16.a5, 16.c
Retained energy	
Current draw	7.1
Power consumption	7.1

Table 18-2 Safety Test Type Versus IEC 601-1 Clause

18.5.2 Enclosure Leakage Current

This test measures enclosure leakages, which is essentially the leakage that a person would be subjected to on touching the device under test. The leakage to ground must be measured from exposed conductive parts of the enclosures, such as connectors, exposed metal, knobs, or shafts, or for fully insulated enclosures from an appropriately sized metal foil. The standard specifies that this test be made with ground open and closed under all possible combinations of open neutral, AC line reversed, external sink voltage reverse polarity, functional earth terminal grounded, and patient lead grounded. Here again, all combinations must be tested. However, if any of the conditions, such as applied parts, is absent, the relevant iterations may be omitted. The enclosure leakage current may not exceed specified limits during the test steps. The allowable limits are detailed in Table 18-3. The schematic is shown in Figure 18-2.

18.5.3 Applied Parts Leakage

Applied parts leakage is the most critical of all safety tests because the patient leads are in direct contact with the patient or in the case of invasive devices, are under the patient's skin, where the resistance is lowest. When applied under the skin, as little as 15 microamps may be fatal. This low current measurement requires a very sensitive and accurate measuring instrument. The

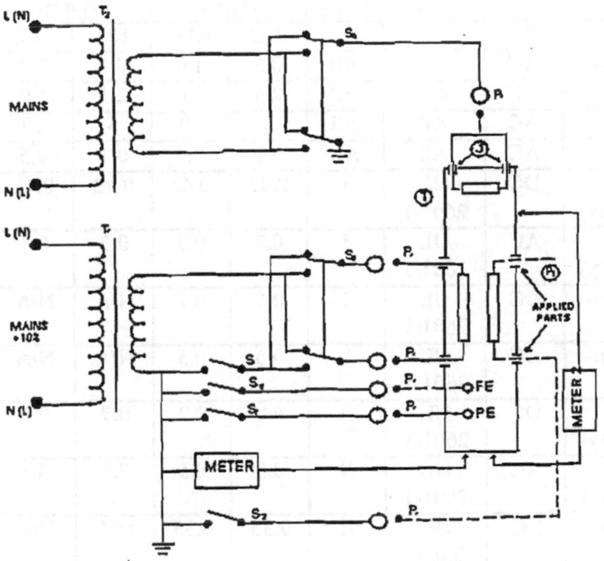

Figure 18-1 Schematic for earth leakage current testing. (From Drefs, 1997)

most complicated and time consuming of all the safety tests due to the sheer number of possible combinations that must be tested are patient lead leakage tests that measure the leakage that could flow through a patient under all the conditions involved when ten or more leads touch a patient and the patient, in turn, touches other nearby objects.

The standard specifies three separate instances in which patient lead leakages should be measured:

- in type B equipment, from all patient connections connected together or with applied parts loaded according to the manufacturer's instructions
- in type BF equipment, from and to all patient connections of a single function of the applied part

Type of Leakage	AC or DC	Std	Class	Allowable Values (milliamps) Applied Part					
				Type B		Type BF		Type CF	
				NC	NFC	NC	NFC	NC	NFC
Earth (general)	AC	All	All	0.5	1.0	0.5	1.0	0.5	1.0
Earth	AC	All	All	2.5	5.0	2.5	5.0	2.5	5.0
Earth	AC	All	All	5	10	5	10	5	10
Enclosure	AC	All	All	0.1	0.5	0.1	0.5	0.1	0.5
Enclosure (patient vicinity)	DC	UL 2601-1	I	0.42	0.42	0.42	0.42	0.42	0.42
Enclosure (patient vicinity)	AC	UL 2601-1	I	0.3	0.3	0.3	0.3	0.3	0.3
Enclosure (non-patient area)	DC	UL 2601-1	I	0.7	0.7	N/A	N/A	N/A	N/A
Enclosure (non-patient area)	AC	UL 2601-1	I	0.5	0.5	N/A	N/A	N/A	N/A
Enclosure (patient vicinity)	DC	UL 2601-1	II	0.7	0.7	0.7	0.7	0.7	0.7
Enclosure (patient vicinity)	AC	UL 2601-1	II	0.5	0.5	0.5	0.5	0.5	0.5
Enclosure (non-patient area)	DC	UL 2601-1	II	0.35	0.35	N/A	N/A	N/A	N/A
Enclosure (non-patient area)	AC	v	II	0.25	0.25	N/A	N/A	N/A	N/A
Patient (mains in SIP or SOP)	AC	All	All	N/A	5.0	N/A	N/A	N/A	N/A
Patient (mains in applied part)	AC	All	All	N/A	N/A	N/A	5.0	N/A	0.05
Patient auxiliary	DC	All	All	0.01	0.05	0.01	0.05	0.01	0.05
Patient auxiliary	AC	All	All	0.1	0.5	0.1	0..5	0.1	0.5

Table 18-3 Limits for Earth-Leakage Current (From Drefs, 1997)

- connected together or with applied parts loaded according to the manufacturer's instructions in type BF equipment, from and to every patient connection in turn.

Additionally, in all types of equipment, the patient auxiliary current must be measured between a single patient connection and all other patient connections connected together.

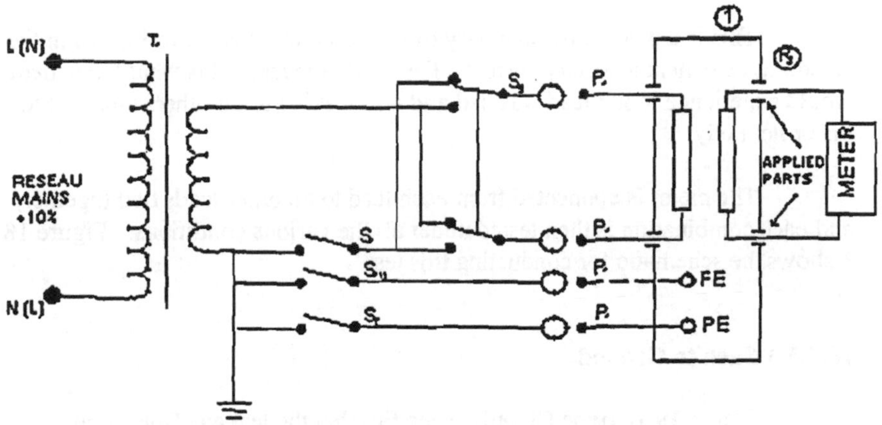

Figure 18-2 Schematic for enclosure leakage current testing. (From Drefs, 1997)

18.5.3.1 All to Ground

The user must measure the total leakage from all of the leads tied together to ground. This configuration simulates what happens when all of the leads are in contact with a patient and the patient touches a grounded object. This is the worst-case summary of the "each to ground" tests. Functional groups can also be tested in this way by disconnecting those leads not included in the group of interest.

The schematic for this test is the same as that for all to ground, but all the leads are tied together rather than kept separate.

18.5.3.2 Each to All Others

This is a worst-case summary of the "each to other" tests known in the standards as patient auxiliary current. The current measured is what the patient would experience if one lead was bad and was leaking to all others attached to his or her body.

The meter is connected from each lead to all other leads tied together, and each combination is then tested under all the various conditions. Figure 18-3 shows the schematic for conducting this test.

18.5.3.3 Each to Ground

Clause 19.1e (type CF only) specifies that the leakage from each applied part to earth must be measured with safety ground closed under all possible combinations of open neutral, AC line reversed, and functional earth terminal grounded, and with safety ground open under all possible combinations of AC line reversed, equipment functional earth grounded, and isolated exposed metal grounded. This simulates the leakage that would flow through a patient who had that lead connected to his or her skin and came in contact with ground.

The "each to ground" test measures the leakage from each individual patient lead to safety ground under various possible conditions. The schematic for the test is shown in Figure 18-4.

18.5.3.4 Sink Each to Ground

The standard specifies that the leakage from each applied part to earth with a sink voltage applied must be measured with line normal and reversed under all possible combinations of external sink voltage reversed, functional earth terminal grounded, and isolated exposed metal grounded to earth.

The "sink each to ground" test measures the leakage from each patient lead to ground in the event that 120 V is present between the lead and ground. This is a worst-case condition. The schematic for the test is shown in Figure 18-5.

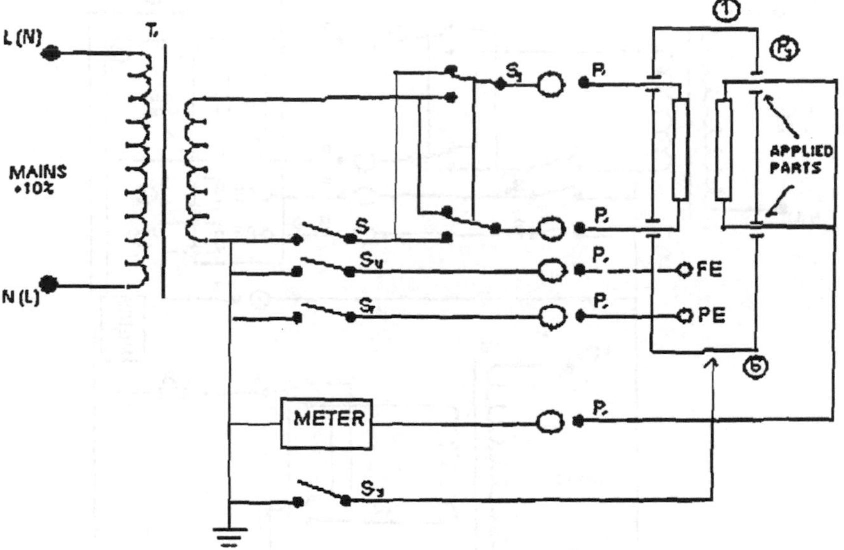

Figure 18-3 Schematic for the each to all others test. (from Drefs, 1997)

18.5.3.5 Sink All to Ground

The standard specifies that the leakage from all applied parts tied together to earth with a sink voltage applied must be measured with line normal and reversed under all possible combinations of external sink voltage reversed, functional earth terminal grounded, and isolated exposed metal grounded to earth. This test measures the leakage from each patient lead to ground in the event that 120 V or 240 V is present between the lead and ground. This is a worse-case condition.

The schematic for this test is the same as that for "sink each to ground" testing, but with all leads tied together.

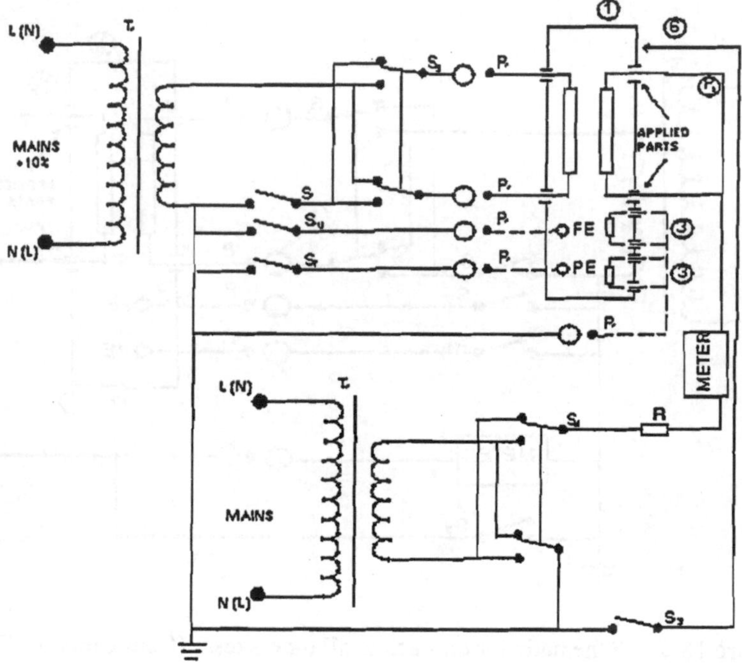

Figure 18-4 Schematic for the each to ground test. (from Drefs, 1997)

18.5.3.6 Each to Probe

For internally powered equipment, the standard specifies that the leakage from each applied part to the enclosure must be measured under normal conditions. If the results are in doubt, the applied parts and live parts are shorted and the leakage is tested again. This represents the leakage that would flow through a patient who touched the equipment enclosure with the patient leads attached to his or her skin.

18.5.3.7 All to Probe

This is a worst-case summary of the "each to probe" tests, used only for internally powered equipment. It measures the leakage from all the leads

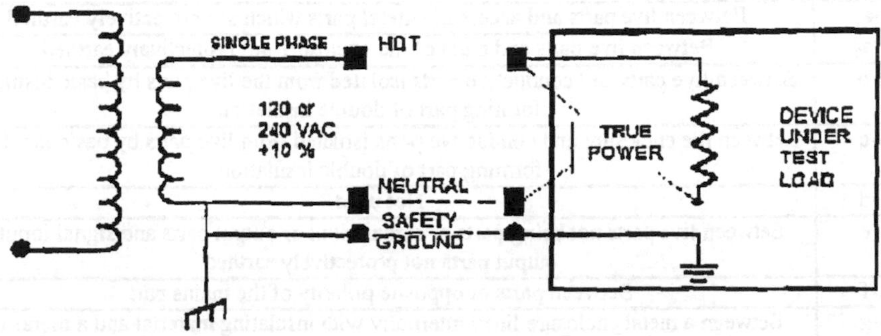

Figure 18-5 Schematic for sink each to ground test. (from Drefs, 1997)

tied together to the enclosure, simulating what would be experienced by a patient who touched the equipment with all the patient leads connected.

18.5.4 Dielectric Withstand

Clause 20 requires that the dielectric strength be investigated between the components listed in Table 18-4. Voltages are applied between the components as listed in Tables 18-5 through 18-7. Notation beginning with *A* are general requirements and those with *B* are particular requirements for equipment with an applied part.

18.5.5 Ground-bond Continuity

Clause 18.f specifies that the safety ground system in the device under test must be tested to ensure that grounded parts of the product are solidly

Notation	Location
A-a_1	Between live parts and accessible metal parts which are protectively earthed
A-a_2	Between live parts and parts of the enclosure not protectively earthed
A-b	Between live parts and conductive parts isolated from the live parts by basic insulation forming part of double insulation
A-c	Between the enclosure and conductive parts isolated from live parts by basic insulation forming part of double insulation
A-d	Not used
A-e	Between live parts not being parts of signal input or output parts and signal input or output parts not protectively earthed
A-f	Between parts of opposite polarity of the mains part
A-g	Between a metal enclosure lined internally with insulating material and a metal foil applied for testing purposes in contact with the inner surface of the lining
A-h	Not used
A-j	Between accessible parts not protectively earthed and likely to become live in the event of a failure of the insulation of the power supply cord, and either metal foil wrapped around the power supply cord inside inlet bushings, cord guards, cord anchorages and the like, or a metal rod having the same diameter as the power supply cord, inserted in its place
A-k	Between, in turn, a signal input part, a signal output part, and accessible parts not protectively earthed
B-a	Between the applied part and live parts
B-b	Between parts of the applied part and/or between applied parts
B-c	Between the applied part and parts not protectively earthed which are isolated from live parts by basic insulation only
B-d	Between an F-type applied part and the enclosure, including signal input and output parts
B-e	Between an F-type applied part and the enclosure where the F-type applied part contains voltages stressing the insulation to the enclosure in normal use including earthing of any part of the applied part
B-f	Not used

Table 18-4 Location of dielectric strength testing.

connected to earth ground through the safety ground conductor. It is also necessary to verify that the chassis and all accessible conductive parts are firmly connected to the safety ground of the product. A current of 25 A or 1.5 times the current consumption of the product, whichever is greater, must be used with a maximum voltage of 6 volts. The resistance should be less than

	Test Voltages for Reference Voltage *U* (volts)					
Notation	U≤50	50<U ≤150	150<U ≤250	250<U≤1,000	1,000<U ≤10.000	10.000<U[2)]
A-a						
Basic Insulation	500	1,000	1,500	2U+1,000	-	-
Supplementary Insulation [2)]	-	2,000	2,500	2U+2,000	-	-
Reinforced Insulation [3)]	-	3,000	4,000	2(2U+1,500)	-	-
A-e	500	1,000	1,500	2U+1,000	-	-
A-f	500	1,000	1,500	2U+1,000	U+2,000	1.20U
A-g	-	1,000	1,500	2U+1,000	U+2,000	1.20U
A-h	-	1,000	1,500	2U+1,000	U+2,000	-
A-j	-	1,000	1,500	2U+1,000	U+2,000	-
A-k	500	1,000	1,500	2U+1,000	U+2,000	1.20U
B-a	500	3,000	1,500	2(2U+1,500)	2(2U+2,500)	-
B-b	1)	1)	1)	1)	1)	1)
B-d	500	1,000	1,500	2U+1,000	U+2,000	-
B-e	1)	1)	1)	1)	1)	1)
B-f	500	3,000	4,000	2(2U+1,500)	2(2U+2,500)	-

1) To be prescribed by particular standards.
2) Unless otherwise prescribed in a particular standard.
3) If applicable, see sub-clause 2.3.

Table 18-5 Test Voltages for Class I Equipment (From IEC 601-1, 1988)

0.1 ohm for detachable cord equipment or 0.2 ohm for permanently attached power cord equipment.

18.5.6 Residual Voltage

The standard requires that the residual voltage present between the supply pins of the power cord plug or between either supply pin and the enclosure, second after disconnection from power, be less than 60 V. If this limit is exceeded, the total energy present must be less than 2 mJ. These tests are designed to ensure that when a piece of equipment is unplugged, the user does not get a shock from inadvertently touching the pins of the poser cord plug

Notation	Test Voltages for Reference Voltage *U* (volts)				
	U≤50	50<U ≤150	150<U ≤250	250<U≤1,000	1,000<U ≤10.000
A-a	500	3,000	4,000	2(2U+1500)	-
A-b	500	1,000	1,500	2U+1000	-
A-c	500	2,000	2,500	2U+2000	U+3,000
A-e	500	3,000	4,000	2(2U+1500)	-
A-f	500	1,000	1,500	2U+1000	U+2,000
A-g	500	2,000	2,500	2U+2000	U+3,000
A-h	500	2,000	2,500	2U+2000	U+3,000
A-j	500	2,000	2,500	2U+2000	U+3,000
A-k	500	3,000	4,000	2(2U+1500)	2(U+2,500)[2)]
B-a	500	3,000	4,000	2(2U+1500)	2(U+2,500)[2)]
B-b	1)	1)	1)	1)	1)
B-c	500	2,000	2,500	2U+2000	1.5U+2,500
B-d	500	2,000	2,500	2U+2000	1.5U+2,500
B-e	1)	1)	1)	1)	1)
B-f	500	3,000	4,000	2(2U+1500)	2(U+2,500)[2)]

1) To be prescribed by particular standards.
2) Unless otherwise prescribed in a particular standard.

Table 18-6 Test Voltages for Class II Equipment (From IEC 601-1, 1988)

immediately after it is disconnected. This voltage is often caused by excess capacitance to ground, which discharges slowly when the power is interrupted.

This is a somewhat complicated test, requiring an instantaneous voltage measurement 1 second after disconnect with no loading during the 1 second interval. Use of a digital scope is not the best option, because it is loaded down during the 1 second interval. It is better to switch in the measurement device after exactly one second and then take the instantaneous peak voltage measurement. This test is done automatically with the BAPCO IEC 601L Safety Tester using only one button.

There are three configurations to check in this test:

B-b	1)
B-d	500
B-e	1)
B-r	500

1) To be prescribed by particular standards.

Table 18-7 Test Voltages for Class III Equipment (From IEC 601-1, 1988)

- hot to neutral
- hot to ground
- neutral to ground.

18.5.7 Accessible-Parts Voltage

The standard specifies that the voltage between accessible parts and earth/safety ground must not exceed 25 V AC or 60 V DC or Peak (no delay used). This ensures that no excessive potential difference exists between the accessible parts and ground during normal operation or after equipment has been de-energized and the access covers are removed. If the unit bears a label specifying a delay time before it may be touched or opened, then this test can be used to verify the label is correct.

18.5.8 Retained Energy

This test is necessary only if the accessible parts voltage measured in the previous test exceeds the 60 V DC or 25 V AC limit. It verifies that there is less than 2mJ of charge stored in the accessible part. To perform this test, you need a millijoule meter, such as the one found in the BAPCO IEC 601 L Universal Safety Tester.

18.5.9 Current Draw

Clause 7.1 specifies that the actual maximum current drawn by the device be compared to the "markings on the equipment." The actual current must be within 10 to 25% (depending on the type of equipment) of the rating on the equipment. This test measures the current that the product under test consumes through the power cord.

With the power turned on, set the AC line polarity to normal. Turn on the product under test. Once it is operating at a steady state as it would in normal use, press the current draw button and read the current in amps on the LCD.

18.5.10 Power Consumption

Clause 7.1 specifies that the user must measure the power the product under test is consuming when operating. The standard requires that this value be compared to the "markings on the equipment" to verify that the power consumption is not more than 10 to 15% higher than the equipment ratings. True power is essential for this measurement because phase shift errors can cause up to 15% variations in the measurement. The equipment controls must be adjusted to maximum output for this measurement to obtain the true maximum, not just the nominal value.

18.6 Proof of Compliance

Knowing why safety tests are necessary, which to perform, and how to perform them, is important, but being able to prove your product's compliance is just as important, especially in the event of a failure in the field or an accident. The only way to prove that you safety tested your device is through testing documentation. You may document it yourself, or pay a third party to do it for you. Either way, you must prove that your medical device was certified to the IEC 601-1 standard.

The best option is to be proactive, now. Make sure your company's devices conform to the standard and are certified to the standard before the deadline arrives. A multi-step approach consists of:

- obtaining a copy of the standard for reference
- getting the test equipment you need to check compliance
- checking your equipment for conformity
- deciding whether to have a third party test lab certify you products, or to self-certify.

These simple steps will enable you to continue shipping your products worldwide and avoid the costly crisis of last-minute certification.

References

Drefs, Martin J., "IEC 601-1 Electrical Safety Testing," in *Compliance Engineering.* Volume XIV, Number 2, March/April, 1997.

Drefs, Martin J., "IEC 601-1 Electrical Safety Testing Part 2: Performing the Tests," in *Compliance Engineering.* Volume XIV, Number 3, May/June, 1997.

International Electrotechnical Commission, *IEC 601-1: Safety of Medical Electrical Equipment, Part 1: General Requirements.* Geneva: International Electrotechnical Commission, 1977.

International Electrotechnical Commission, *IEC 601-1: Medical Electrical Equipment, Part 1: General Requirements for Safety.* Geneva: International Electrotechnical Commission, 1988.

International Electrotechnical Commission, *IEC 601-1-1: Safety of Medical Electrical Equipment, Part 1: General Requirements for Safety 1. Collateral Standard: Safety Requirements for Medical Electrical Systems.* Geneva: International Electrotechnical Commission, 1992.

Chapter 19

IEC 601-1 Requirements/Compliance

This general standard contains requirements on safety which are generally applicable to medical electrical equipment. For certain types of equipment, these requirements may have to be supplemented or modified by the special requirements of a particular standard. Where particular standards exist, the general standard is not to be used alone.

Requirements of this standard are grouped according to the following categories:

- Safety Requirements
- Protection Against Electric Shock Hazards
- Protection Against Mechanical Hazards
- Protection Against Hazards from Unwanted or Excessive Radiation
- Protection Against Hazards of Explosions in Medically Used Rooms
- Protection Against Excessive Temperatures, Fire, and Other Hazards, such as Human Errors
- Accuracy of Operating Data and Protection Against Incorrect Output

- Fault Conditions Causing Overheating and/or Mechanical Damage
- Constructional Requirements.

Not every requirement or detail from the standard is covered here. Each section covers the mains points within the section. The reader is referred to the document itself to obtain the details of the requirements.

19.1 General Requirements

19.1.1 Requirements

Clause 3 — A system after installation or subsequent modification must not cause a safety hazard for the patient, the operator, or surroundings.

Clause 4 — After installation or subsequent modification, the system must be in compliance with the requirements of this standard.

Clause 6 — Where in the accompanying documents a warning is given related to a particular safety hazard from a non-medical, a symbol must be provided on that particular non-medical electrical equipment or on a particular part of that equipment.

A system after installation or subsequent modification must be accompanied by documents containing all data necessary for safe and reliable use.

19.1.2 Compliance

Clause 3 — Compliance is checked by inspection of appropriate documents or certificates.

Clause 4 — Compliance is checked by inspection, testing, or analysis.

Clause 6 — Compliance is checked by inspection.

19.2 Environmental Conditions

19.2.1 Requirements

Unless otherwise stated by the manufacturer, equipment must be capable, while packaged for transport or storage, of being exposed for a period not exceeding 15 weeks to environmental conditions not outside the following ranges:

- an ambient temperature range of -40°C to +70°C
- a relative humidity range of 10% to 100%, including condensation
- an atmospheric pressure of 500 hPa to 1060 hPa.

Equipment must comply with all the requirements of this standard when operated in normal use under the least favorable combination of the following conditions:

- an ambient temperature range of +10°C to +40°C
- a relative humidity range of 30% to 75%, including condensation
- an atmospheric pressure of 700 hPa to 1060 hPa.
- a temperature of the water at the inlet of water-cooled equipment not higher than 25°C.

19.2.2 Compliance

Compliance is checked by testing and analysis.

19.3 Protection Against Electric Shock Hazards

19.3.1 Requirements

Clause 13 Equipment must be so designed that the risk of electric shock in normal use and in single fault condition is obviated as far as practicable.

Clause 14 For protection against electric shock, at least the mains part of equipment must be provided in addition to the basic insulation with an additional protection according to the requirements of Class I, II, or III equipment.

In the case of equipment specified for power supply from an external d.c. power source, not hazard to patient, user, or equipment must develop when a connection with the wrong polarity is made.

The mains part must be isolated from accessible conductive parts. If this isolation is accomplished by basic insulation only, then, in addition to the conductors for connection to the battery system, a separate protective earth conductor must be provided.

In Class II equipment, capacitors must not be connected between parts which carry mains voltage and accessible conductive parts, nor shall the conductive enclosure of such capacitors or an enclosure of such capacitors made of insulating material and providing only basic insulation, be secured directly to accessible conductive parts.

For Class III equipment, the safety extra-low voltage must be restricted to medical safety extra-low voltage.

Clause 15

Circuits in a medical safety extra-low voltage part must not be connected to circuits with voltages above medical safety extra-low voltage.

All insulation in a medical safety extra-low voltage part must be designed for a test voltage of 500 V.

Equipment intended to be connected to the supply by means of a plug must be so designed that one second after disconnection of the plug, the voltage between the supply pins of the plug or between either supply pin and body of the equipment does not exceed 50 V. Capacitors or circuit parts connected to them, which become accessible after equipment has been de-energized and access covers have been removed immediately thereafter, must not have a residual voltage exceeding 50 V, or, if this value is exceeded, must not have a residual energy exceeding 2 mJ.

Clause 16 Equipment must be so constructed and enclosed that there is adequate protection against accidental contact with live parts and, for Class II equipment, with conductive parts separated from live parts by basic insulation only.

Any opening in a top cover of an enclosure must be so positioned or dimensioned that accessibility of live parts by means of a freely and vertically suspended test rod with a diameter of 4 mm and a length of 100 mm, penetrating up to its length, is prevented.

Shafts of actuating parts which are accessible after the removal of handles, knobs, levers, and the like must not be live.

Parts within the enclosure of equipment with a circuit voltage exceeding 24 V which cannot be disconnected from the supply by an external mains switch or a plug device that is accessible at all times must be protected against accidental contact even after opening of the enclosure by additional coverings or, in the case of a spatially separated arrangement, must still be marked clearly as *live*.

Enclosures, protecting against contact with live parts must be removable only with the aid of a tool or, alternatively, an automatic device must make these parts not live when the enclosure is opened or removed

Openings for the adjustment of pre-set controls which may be adjusted by the user in normal use by using a tool must be so designed that the tool used for adjustment is not able to touch inside the opening by live parts or conductive parts of Class II equipment separated from the mains part by basic insulation only.

Equipment must be so constructed as to prevent the penetration from the table or floor of foreign objects which might have an adverse effect on the safety of the equipment.

If an enclosure has openings in the bottom surface, all live parts must be at least at a distance of 6 mm from the supporting surface, measured vertically through any opening.

Clause 17

An applied part must be separated from live parts of the equipment, particularly from the mains part. Deterioration of parts by use and aging must be taken into account.

In case of a single fault condition or in case of defects of thermionic valves and/or semiconductors, wire rupture, or disconnection of a component in other parts, the applied parts must not produce a patient leakage current exceeding the allowable value for single fault conditions (see Table 19-1).

Accessible conductive parts in Class II and III equipment and in equipment with an internal electrical power source must not be connected to an applied part.

Hand-held flexible shafts of Class I equipment must be isolated from the motor shaft by supplementary insulation.

Accessible conductive parts driven by an electric motor of Class I protection and which during normal use are likely to come into direct contact with a user or patient, and which cannot be protectively earthed in accordance with the requirements of Clause 18

Current Path	Type B		Type BF		Type CF	
	NC	SFC	NC	SFC	NC	SFC
Earth leakage current	0.5	1	0.5	1	0.5	1
Earth leakage current for equipment according to notes 2 and 4.	2,5	5	2.5	5	2.5	5
Earth leakage current for equipment according to note 3	5	10	5	10	5	10
Enclosure leakage current	0.1	0.5	0.1	0.5	0.1	0.5
Patient leakage current	0.1	0.5	0.1	0.5	0.01	0.05
Patient leakage current (mains voltage on the signal input part and signal output part)	-	5	-	-	-	-
Patient leakage current (mains voltage on the applied part)	-	-	-	5	-	0.05
Patient auxiliary current dc	0.01	0.5	0.01	0.05	0.01	0.05
ac	0.1	0.5	0.1	0.5	0.01	0.05

NC = normal condition
SFC = single fault condition

Note 1: the only single fault condition for the earth leakage current is the interruption of one supply conductor at a time.

Note 2: equipment which has no protectively earthed accessible parts and no means for the protective earthing of other equipment and which complies with the requirements for the enclosure leakage current and for the patient leakage current.

Note 3: equipment specified to be permanently installed with a protective earth Conductor which is electrically so connected that the connection can only be loosened with the aid of a tool and which is so fastened or otherwise so secured mechanically at a specific location that it can only be moved after the use of a tool.

Note 4: mobile X-ray equipment and mobile equipment with mineral insulation.

Table 19-1 Allowable Values of Continuous Leakage and Patient Auxiliary Currents, in Milliamperes (from IEC 601-1-1, 1988)

and 58, must be isolated from the motor shaft by at least supplementary insulation capable of withstanding the dielectric strength test appropriate to the rated voltage of the motor and having adequate mechanical strength.

Accessible non-conductive surfaces of Class I equipment must be so constructed that a metal foil applied in contact with such a surface must not become live in the case of breakdown of a basic insulation.

Clause 18

Generally, accessible conductive parts of Class I equipment must be connected permanently and with sufficiently low impedance to the protective earth terminal.

A protective earth conductor must not be fused.

The insulation of a protective earth conductor must be colored according to sub-clause 6.5.

Functional earth terminals must not be used to provide protective earthing.

The protective earth terminal or contact must be connected to an external protective system by either a protective earth conductor in a flexible supply cable or cord and an appropriate plug or a fixed and permanently installed protective earth conductor.

A protective earth pathway must not be used to carry functional events.

Equipment having a conductive enclosure or an enclosure with an accessible conductive part and:

- of Class II with an applied part
- of Class III with an applied part
- with an internal electrical power source and an applied part, or
- of Type CF

must be provided with a facility for the connection of a potential equalization conductor if such equipment

is also specified for use in medically used rooms where potential equalization is required.
The facility for the connection must be readily accessible, must be such that accidental loosening is prevented in normal use and must be such that the potential equalization conductor can be detached from the equipment when the equipment is used outside those medically used rooms where potential equalization is required.

The potential equalization conductor must not be included in the power supply cable or cord of the equipment.

Any potential equalization conductor must be identified throughout its length by green/yellow colored insulation.

For equipment without a flexible supply cable or cord, the resistance between the protective earth terminal and any other part which is connected to it for protective purposes must not exceed 0.1 Ω.

For equipment with a detachable supply cable or cord, the resistance between the protective contact in the appliance inlet and any other part which is connected to it for protective purposes must not exceed 0.1 Ω.

For equipment with a non-detachable flexible supply cable or cord, the resistance between the protective contact in the mains plug and any other part which is connected to it for protective purposes must not exceed 0.2 Ω.

The maximum permitted resistance of the protective earthing connection for accessories connected to equipment, if exceeding 0.1 Ω, must be determined according to:

$$R_{PE} \leq (I_{ENCL}/I_V)R_T$$

where:

R_{PE} = resistance of protective earth connection in ohms

I_{ENCL} = allowable value of the enclosure leakage current in single fault conditions in milliamperes

I_V = maximum continuous single fault current in amperes

R_T = test resistance in kilo-ohms.

Where an additional protective earth conductor is used, any connector in the additional protective earth conductor of the equipment, if provided as a lead separate from the power supply cord, must be provided with a suitable, retaining device to prevent inadvertent disconnection from the equipment during normal use.

An additional protective earth conductor must comply at least with the requirements for the normal protective earth conductor.

Clause 19

The electrical insulation of equipment providing protection against electric shock must have such a quality that the currents flowing through it are limited to the specified values.

The specified values of the continuous earth leakage current, the enclosed leakage current, the patient leakage current, and the patient auxiliary current apply in any combination of the following conditions:

- both at operating temperature and following the humidity preconditioning treatment
- in normal condition and in the specified single fault conditions
- with equipment energized in stand-by condition and fully operating and with

any switch in the mains part in any position

- with the highest rated supply frequency
- with a supply equal to 110% of the highest rated mains voltage.

In normal condition, the allowable enclosure leakage current from or between parts of the system within the patient environment must not exceed 0.1 mA.

In the event of the interruption of any non-permanently installed protective earth conductor in the allowable enclosure, leakage current from or between parts of a system within the patient environment must not exceed 0.5 mA.

In normal condition, the patient leakage current must not exceed 0.1 mA for type B and BF equipment and 0.01 mA for type CF equipment.

Allowable values for leakage current have been listed in Table 19-1.

Clause 20 The dielectric strength must be tested between those parts listed in Table 18-4

The dielectric strength of the electrical insulation at the operating temperature as well as following humidity preconditioning treatment and after any required sterilization procedure, if applicable, must be sufficient to withstand the test voltages as listed in Tables 18-5 through 18-7.

19.3.2 Compliance

Clause 13 Compliance is checked by inspection, testing, or analysis.

Clause 14 Compliance is checked by inspection, testing, or analysis.

Clause 15 Compliance is checked by inspection, testing, or analysis.

Clause 16 Compliance is checked by inspection and by insertion through the opening of a metal test rod with a diameter of 4 mm and a length of 100 mm in every possible position with a force of 10 newtons.

Clause 17 Compliance is checked by inspection, testing, or analysis.

Clause 18 Compliance is checked by inspection and measurement.

Clause 19 Compliance is checked by inspection, testing, or analysis.

Clause 20 Compliance is checked by inspection, testing, or analysis.

Protection against electric shock caused by currents not resulting from the specified physical phenomena of the equipment is obtained by:

- prevention of contact between the body of the patient, the user, or a third person and parts which are live or may become live by means of enclosing, guarding, or mounting the parts in inaccessible locations
- restriction of voltages on or currents from parts which may be touched intentionally or unintentionally by the patient, user, or a third person.

The requirement for prevention of penetration of foreign objects is satisfied:

- for equipment intended to be placed on a table, if the equipment is provided with legs at least 10 mm high

- for equipment intended to be placed on the floor, if the legs of the equipment are at least 20 mm high.

19.4 Protection Against Mechanical Hazards

19.4.1 Requirements

Clause 21 Enclosures, including any access covers forming part of them, with all components thereon, must have sufficient strength and rigidity.

Equipment parts serving for support and/or immobilization of patients must be designed and manufactured so as to minimize the risk of physical injuries and of accidental loosening of fixings.

Equipment or equipment parts which are hand held during normal use must not present a safety hazard as a result of a free fall from a height of 1 meter on to a hard surface.

Portable and mobile equipment must withstand the stresses caused by rough handling.

Clause 22 Moving parts which do not need to be exposed for the operation of equipment and which, if exposed, constitute a safety hazard must 1) in the case of transportable equipment, be provided with adequate guards which must form an integral part of the equipment, or 2) in the case of stationary equipment, be similarly guarded unless installation instructions provided by the require that such guarding or equivalent protection will be separately provided.

Parts subject to mechanical wear likely to result in a safety hazard must be accessible for inspection.

When in a system, movement of equipment or equipment parts may cause a safety hazard, the system must be provided with a protective means, such as an emergency stopping device.

Clause 23 — Rough surfaces, sharp corners, and edges which may cause injury or damage must be avoided or covered.

Clause 24 — Equipment must either not overbalance during normal use when tilted through an angle of 10°.

Clause 25 — Where expelled parts could constitute a safety Hazard, protective means must be provided.

Clause 26 — Not used.

Clause 27 — Not used.

Clause 28 — Where the integrity of a suspension depends on parts, such as springs, which may, due to their manufacturing process, have hidden defects, a safety device must be provided, unless excess travel in the event of a breakdown is limited.

If a safety device is not provided:

- the total load must not exceed the safe working load
- where it is unlikely that supporting characteristics will be impaired by wear, corrosion, material fatigue or aging, the safety factor of all supporting parts must not be less than 4
- where impairment by wear, corrosion, material fatigue, or aging is expected, relevant supporting parts must have a safety factor not less than 8
- where metal, having a specific elongation at break of less than 5%, is used in supporting components, the safety factors given above must be multiplied by 1.5.
- sheaves, sprockets, bandwheels, and guides must be so designed and constructed that the safety factors listed in this clause must be maintained for a

specified minimum life until replacement of the ropes, chains, and bands.

19.4.2 Compliance

Clause 21	Compliance is checked by inspection, testing, or analysis.
Clause 22	Compliance is checked by inspection.
Clause 23	Compliance is checked by inspection.
Clause 24	Compliance is checked by inspection, testing, or analysis.
Clause 25	Compliance is checked by inspection.
Clause 28	Compliance is checked by inspection of the design data and any maintenance instructions.

19.5 Protection Against Hazards from Unwanted or Excessive Radiation

19.5.1 Requirements

Radiation from medical electrical equipment intended for application to patients for diagnostic or therapeutic purpose, under medical supervision, may exceed limits normally accepted for the population as a whole.

Adequate provision must be made to protect the patient, operator, and other persons and sensitive devices in the vicinity of the equipment from unwanted or excessive radiation from the equipment.

19.5.2 Compliance

Compliance is checked by measurement of exposure or exposure rate with a radiation detector suitable for the energy of the emitted radiation.

19.6 Protection Against Hazards of Ignition of Flammable Anesthetic Mixtures

19.6.1 Requirements

Equipment, equipment parts, or components must not ignite flammable anesthetic mixtures with air in normal use and normal condition.

Equipment, equipment parts, or components must not ignite flammable anesthetic mixtures with oxygen or nitrous oxide in normal use and in the event of any applicable single fault condition.

Parts or components of equipment which operate in a flammable anesthetic mixture with oxygen or nitrous oxide must be supplied from a source which is isolated from earth by at least basic insulation and from live parts by double or reinforced insulation.

Equipment, equipment parts, and components which heat a flammable anesthetic mixture with oxygen or nitrous oxide must be provided with a non-self-resetting thermal cut-out, as an additional protection against overheating.

The current-carrying part of the heating element must not be in direct contact with the flammable anesthetic mixture with oxygen or nitrous oxide.

19.6.2 Compliance

Compliance is checked by inspection, testing, measurement, or analysis.

Equipment, equipment parts, or components not producing sparks and not producing operating temperatures of surfaces in contact with gas mixtures in normal use and normal condition, exceeding 150°C in the case of restricted vertical air circulation by convection, or exceeding 200°C in the case of unrestricted vertical air circulation, if measured at an ambient temperature of 25°C, are considered to comply with the requirements of this section.

19.7 Protection Against Excessive Temperatures and Other Safety Hazards

19.7.1 Requirements

Applied parts of equipment not intended to supply heat to a patient must not have surface temperatures exceeding 41°C.

Guards intended to prevent contact with hot accessible surfaces must be removable only with the aid of a tool.

The construction of equipment must ensure a sufficient degree of protection against safety hazards caused by overflow, spillage, leakage, humidity, ingress of liquids, cleaning, sterilization, and disinfection.

The maximum pressure to which a part can be subjected in normal or abnormal operation must not exceed the maximum permissible working pressure for the part.

Thermal cut-outs and over-current releases with automatic resetting must not be used if they may cause a safety hazard by such resetting.

Means must be provided to allow the mechanical constraints on a patient to be removed in the event of failure of the supply mains.

A system must be so designed that an interruption and restoration of the power supply must not result in a safety hazard other than interruption of its intended function.

19.7.2 Compliance

Compliance is checked by inspection, testing, or analysis.

19.8 Accuracy of Operating Data and Protection Against Hazardous Output

19.8.1 Requirements

If the control range of equipment is such that the delivered output in a part of the range considerably differs from the output which is regarded as non-hazardous, means must be provided that prevent such a setting or which indicate to the operator that the selected setting is in excess of a safety limit.

Any equipment delivering energy or substances to a patient must indicate the possible hazardous output, preferably as a pre-indication.

Where equipment is a multi-purpose unit designed for providing both low-intensity and high-intensity outputs for different treatments, appropriate steps must be taken to minimize the possibility of a high intensity output being selected accidentally.

19.8.2 Compliance

Compliance is checked by inspection.

19.9 Abnormal Operation and Fault Conditions

19.9.1 Requirements

Equipment must be so designed and manufactured that even in single fault conditions, no safety hazard exists.

19.9.2 Compliance

Compliance is checked by inspection, testing, or analysis.

19.10 Constructional Requirements

19.10.1 Requirements

Ratings of components must not conflict with the conditions of use in equipment.

All components in the mains part and in the applied part must be marked or otherwise identified so that their ratings can be ascertained.

Components, the unwanted movement of which could result in a safety hazard, must be mounted securely to prevent such movement.

Conductors and connectors must be so secured and/or insulated that accidental detachment must not result in a safety hazard.

Design and construction of electrical, hydraulic, pneumatic, and gas connection terminals and connectors must be such that incorrect connection of accessible connectors, removable without the use of a tool, must be prevented where a safety hazard may be caused.

Detachable flexible cords used for interconnection of different parts of equipment must be provided with means for connection such that accessible metal parts cannot become live when a connection is loosened or broken due to the disengagement of one or the connecting means.

Housings containing batteries from which gases can escape during charging or discharging must be ventilated to minimize the risk of accumulation and ignition.

Plugs for connection of patient circuit leads must be so designed that they cannot be connected to other outlets on the same system, unless it can be proven that no safety hazard can result.

The protective earth conductor connection must be made in such a way that the removal of any single item of equipment in the system will not interrupt the protective earth conductor connection to any part of the system, without at the same time disconnecting the supply of electric energy from that part.

Conductors which connect different item of equipment within a system must be protected against the effects of short-circuiting and overload and be protected against mechanical damage.

Mains supply transformers used in medical electrical equipment must be protected against overheating of basic insulation, supplementary insulation, and reinforced insulation in the event of short-circuit or overload on any output windings.

19.10.2 Compliance

Compliance is checked by inspection, testing, or analysis.

References

International Electrotechnical Commission, *IEC 601-1: Medical Electrical Equipment, Part 1: General Requirements for Safety.* Geneva: International Electrotechnical Commission, 1988.

International Electrotechnical Commission, *IEC 601-1-1: Safety of Medical Electrical Equipment, Part 1: General Requirements for Safety 1. Collateral Standard: Safety Requirements for Medical Electrical Systems.* Geneva: International Electrotechnical Commission, 1992.

Section 4

Regulation

Chapter 20

The Medical Devices Directives

The Medical Devices Directives are a complicated set of directives with device classification, conformity assessment procedures, and rules. Medical manufacturers need to decide which one best suits their company and product, and which is the most cost effective.

The European Community's program on the Completion of the Internal Market has, as the primary objective for medical devices, to ensure Community-wide free circulation of products. The only means to establish such free circulation, in view of quite divergent national systems, regulations governing medical devices, and existing trade barriers, was to adopt legislation for the Community, by which the health and safety of patients, users and third persons would be ensured through a harmonized set of device-related protection requirements. Devices meeting the requirements and sold to members of the Community are identified by means of a CE mark.

The Active Implantable Medical Devices Directive adopted by the Community legislature in 1990 and the Medical Devices Directive in 1993 cover more than 80% of medical devices for use with human beings. After a period of transition, i.e., a period during which the laws implementing a directive co-exist with pre-existing national laws, these directives exhaustively govern the conditions for placing medical devices on the market. Through the agreements in the European Economic Area (EEA), the relevant requirements and procedures are the same for all European Community (EC) member states and European Free Trade Association (EFTA) countries that belong to the EEA, an economic area comprising more than 380 million people.

20.1 History

The Medical Devices Directive 93/42/EEC came into effect on January 1, 1995. It will be enforced beginning June 15, 1998. Until that time, manufacturers can either comply with individual national regulations or meet the requirements of the Medical Devices Directive (MDD) and CE mark its product. After June 15, 1998, however, the manufacturer must meet the requirements of the MDD.

20.2 General Provisions

The Medical Devices Directive applies to all devices which are principally intended for one of the following purposes:

- diagnosis
- prevention monitoring
- treatment or alleviation of disease
- injury/replacement/modification of the anatomy.

It specifically excludes active implantable devices and in-vitro diagnostic devices which are covered by their own directives, but it does include any electronic apparatus, such as personal computers and their software, which are principally used for medical purposes.

Like all new approach directives, the MDD requires that a medical product complies with a set of essential requirements relating to performance, health, and safety. These requirements, focusing on the safety aspects of the design and construction, cover issues such as chemical, physical, and biological properties, infection, and microbial contamination, EMC, radiation, mechanical, thermal, and electrical risks. Again, as in the other directives, standards will be available to enable compliance with the requirements to be demonstrated. However, compliance with the standards themselves will not be mandatory. Medical device makers have the following legal obligations:

- the product must meet the essential requirements defined in Annex I of the Directive, where applicable

- the manufacturer must demonstrate this compliance by following one of the conformity assessment procedures laid down in Article 11 and Annexes II - VII.

20.3 Definition of a Medical Device

The various medical device directives define a medical device as:

"any instrument, appliance, apparatus, material or other article, whether used alone or in combination, including the software necessary for its proper application, intended by the manufacturer to be used for human beings for the purpose of:

- diagnosis, prevention, monitoring, treatment or alleviation of disease;
- diagnosis, monitoring, alleviation of or compensation for an injury or handicap;
- investigation, replacement or modification of the anatomy or of a physiological process;
- control of conception;

and which does not achieve its principal intended action in or on the human body by pharmacological, immunological, or metabolic means, but which may be assisted in its function by such means."

One important feature of the definition is that it emphasizes the "intended use" of the device and its "principal intended action." This use of the term *intended* gives manufacturers of certain products some opportunity to include or exclude their product from the scope of the particular directive.

Another important feature of the definition is the inclusion of the term *software*. The software definition will probably be given further interpretation, but is currently interpreted to mean that 1) software intended to control the function of a device is a medical device, 2) software for patient records or other administrative purposes is not a device, 3) software which is built into a device, e.g., software in an electrocardiographic monitor used to drive a display, is clearly an integral part of the medical device, and 4) a software update sold by the manufacturer, or a variation sold by a software house, is a medical device in its own right.

20.4 Classification of Medical Products

There are four main categories for medical devices:

- Class I
- Class IIa
- Class IIb
- Class III.

The classification system is discussed in Annex IX, Section III of the Medical Devices Directive. Remember, it is the intended purpose of the device and not the particular technical characteristics that determines the class of the product. Class I represents the lowest risk products, generally those which do not make contact with the patient. Class III, on the other hand, imposes the greatest risk to safety, and thus requires more stringent conformity requirements.

Class I includes general, unpowered or non-active devices which do not penetrate the body or non-surgically invasive devices for transient use (less than 60 minutes). Some low risk powered (active) devices for patient support or examination are also included.

Class IIa includes non-hazardous active therapeutic and diagnostic devices. Low risk surgically invasive devices for transient use or short term use (up to 30 days) are also included.

Class IIb includes potentially hazardous active therapeutic and diagnostic devices. Also included are higher risk surgically invasive devices for transient or short term use and surgically invasive devices for long term or implantable (non-active) use (not more than 30 days).

Class III includes all devices which make contact with the heart and central circulatory system or central nervous system, as well as all long term invasive or implantable devices which have biological effect on the body or are absorbed into it.

20.5 Conformity Assessment Requirements

A manufacturer can look at Article 11 of the Medical Devices Directive to determine which route to follow to conformity. There is a requirement to assess both the product and the manufacturer's ability to produce consistently compliant products. There is therefore heavy emphasis on Quality Assurance. The routes to conformity depend on the classification of the product.

20.5.1 Class I Products

These follow the Declaration of Conformity procedure laid out in Annex VII. This is basically self certification, where the manufacturer declares that the product meets the essential requirements. There is a presumption of compliance where harmonized standards are met. No Notified Body involvement is required, except in the case of sterile products and measuring devices.

20.5.2 Class IIa Products

Here the manufacturer's declaration must be supported by a Notified Body Conformity Assessment. This may, at the manufacturer's choice, consist of an audit of the production QA system laid out in Annex V, or an audit of final inspection and test laid out in Annex VI, or an examination and test of product samples laid out in Annex IV. Alternately, the manufacturer may elect to follow the full QA procedure laid down in Annex II, with the exception of Clause 4 which is not applicable, which involves an audit of the QA system by a Notified Body.

20.5.3 Class IIb Products

For these, the declaration must be supported by an EC Type Examination by a Notified Body, as laid down in Annex III, together with either an audit of the production QA system laid out in Annex V, or an examination and test of product samples laid out in Annex IV. Alternately, the manufacturer may elect to follow the full QA procedure laid down in Annex II, with the exception of Clause 4 which is not applicable, which involves an audit of the QA system by a Notified Body.

20.5.4 Class III Products

The choice is between an EC Type Examination by a Notified Body as laid down in Annex III, together with either an audit of the production QA system laid out in Annex V, or an examination and test of product samples laid out in Annex IV. Alternately, the manufacturer may elect to follow the full QA procedure laid down in Annex II which involves an audit of the QA system by a Notified Body. Clause 4 is applicable and requires a design dossier to be prepared for the product. This dossier is subject to examination by a Notified Body.

20.6 The Medical Devices Directives Process

The process of meeting the requirements of the Medical Devices Directives is a multi-step approach, involving the following activities:

- analyze the device to determine which directive is applicable
- identify the applicable Essential Requirements List
- identify any corresponding Harmonized Standards
- confirm that the device meets the Essential Requirements/Harmonized Standards and document the evidence
- classify the device
- decide on the appropriate conformity assessment procedure
- identify and choose a Notified Body
- obtain conformity certifications for the device
- establish a Declaration of Conformity
- apply for the CE mark.

This process does not necessarily occur in a serial manner, but iterations may occur throughout the cycle. Each activity in the process will be examined in detail.

20.7 Conclusion

Compliance with the new EC Directives will imply major changes for medical device manufacturers. Such changes relate to the requirements to be met in view of the design and manufacture of medical devices as well as to the procedures to be followed by manufacturers prior to and after placing medical devices on the European market. Manufacturers who wish to market medical devices in western Europe are therefore faced with a quite far-reaching and rather complex decision-making process.

References

The Active Implantable Medical Devices Directive. 90/385/EEC, 20 June, 1990.

The Medical Devices Directive. 93/42/EEC, 14 June, 1993.

Draft Proposal for a Council Directive on In Vitro Diagnostic Medical Devices, Working Document. III/D/4181/93, April, 1993.

Fries, R.C. and M. Graber, "Designing Medical Devices for Conformance with Harmonized Standards," *Biomedical Instrumentation & Technology*. Volume 29, Number 4, July/August, 1995.

Fries, Richard C., *Reliable Design of Medical Devices.* New York: Marcel Dekker, Inc., 1997.

Higson, G.R., *The Medical Devices Directive-A Manufacturer's Handbook.* Brussels: Medical Technology Consultants Europe Ltd., 1993.

SWBC, Organization for the European Conformity of Products, *CE-Mark: The New European Legislation for Products.* Milwaukee, WI: ASQC Quality Press, 1996.

Chapter 21

The Medical Devices Directives Requirements and Compliance

The requirements do not necessarily occur in a serial manner, as iterations may occur throughout the cycle.

21.1 Requirements

Each manufacturer must analyze the device to determine which directive is applicable.

Each manufacturer must identify the applicable Essentials Requirements List.

Each manufacturer must identify any corresponding Harmonized Standards.

Each manufacturer must confirm that the device meets the Essential Requirements/Harmonized Standards and document the evidence.

Each manufacturer must classify the device.

Each manufacturer must decide on the appropriate conformity assessment procedure.

Each manufacturer must identify and choose a notified body.

Each manufacturer must obtain conformity certifications for the device.

Each manufacturer must establish a Declaration of Conformity.

Each manufacturer must apply for the CE mark.

21.2 Compliance

21.2.1 Choosing the Appropriate Directive

Because of the diversity of current national medical device regulations, the European Commission decided that totally new Community legislation covering all medical devices was needed. Software or a medical device containing software may be subject to the requirements of the Active Implantable Medical Devices Directive or the Medical Devices Directive.

Three directives are envisaged to cover the entire field of medical devices:

Active Implantable Medical Devices Directive (AIMDD)

This directive applies to a medical device which depends on a source of electrical energy or any source of power other than that directly generated by the human body or gravity, which is intended to be totally or partially introduced, surgically or medically, into the human body or by medical intervention into a natural orifice, and which is intended to remain after the procedure.

This directive was adopted in June, 1990, implemented in January, 1993 and the transition period ended January, 1995.

Medical Devices Directive (MDD)

This directive applies to all medical devices and accessories, unless they are covered by the Active Implantable Medical Devices Directive or the In Vitro Diagnostic Medical Devices Directive.

This directive applies to all medical devices and accessories, unless they are covered by the Active Implantable Medical Devices Directive or the In Vitro Diagnostic Medical Devices Directive.

This directive was adopted in June, 1993, was implemented in January, 1995 and the transition period ends June, 1998.

In Vitro Diagnostic Medical Devices Directive (IVDMDD)

This directive applies to any medical device that is a reagent, reagent product, calibrator, control kit, instrument, equipment or system intended to be used in vitro for the examination of samples derived from the human body for the purpose of providing information concerning a physiological state of health or disease or congenital abnormality, or to determine the safety and compatibility with potential recipients. This directive is currently in preparation.

21.2.2 Identifying the Applicable Essential Requirements

The major legal responsibility the directives place on the manufacturer of a medical device requires the device meet the Essential Requirements set out in Annex I of the directive which applies to them, taking into account the intended purpose of the device. The Essential Requirements are written in the form of 1) general requirements which always apply and 2) particular requirements, only some of which apply to any particular device.

The general requirements for the Essential Requirements List take the following form:

- the device must be safe. Any risk must be acceptable in relation to the benefits offered by the device.
- the device must be designed in such a manner that risk is eliminated or protected against.
- the device must perform in accordance with the manufacturer's specifications.
- the safety and performance must be maintained throughout the indicated lifetime of the device.
- the safety and performance of the device must not be affected by normal conditions of transport and storage.
- any side effects must be acceptable in relation to the benefits offered.

The particular requirements for the Essential Requirements List address the following topics:

- chemical, physical, and biological properties
- infection and microbial contamination
- construction and environmental properties
- devices with a measuring function
- protection against radiation
- requirements for devices connected to or equipped with an energy source
- protection against electrical risks
- protection against mechanical and thermal risks
- protection against the risks posed to the patient by energy supplies or substances
- information supplied by the manufacturer.

The easiest method of ensuring the Essential Requirements are met is to establish a checklist of the Essential Requirements from Appendix I of the appropriate directive, which then forms the basis of the technical dossier. Figure 21-1 is an example of an Essential Requirements checklist.

The Essential Requirements checklist includes 1) a statement of the Essential Requirements, 2) an indication of the applicability of the Essential Requirements to a particular device, 3) a list of the standards used to address the Essential Requirements, 4) the activity that addresses the Essential Requirements, 5) the clause(s) in the standard detailing the applicable test for the particular Essential Requirement, 6) an indication of whether the device passed/or failed the test, and 7) a statement of the location of the test documentation or certificates.

21.2.3 Identification of Corresponding Harmonized Standards

A "harmonized" standard is a standard produced under a mandate from the European Commission by one of the European standardization bodies, such as CEN (the European Committee for Standardization) or CENELEC (the European Committee for Electrotechnical Standardization),

equirements	A or N/A	Standards	Activity	Test Clause	Pass/Fail
al Requirements					
levice must be designed and ed in such a way that, when the conditions and for the ntended, they will not e the clinical condition or the atients, users, and where , other persons. The risks with devices must be reduced ptable level compatible with a of protection for health and	A	Internal	Hazard Analysis Safety review		
solutions adopted by the rer for the design and on of the devices must comply y principles and also take into e generally acknowledged state	A	Internal	Specification reviews Design reviews Safety review		
devices must achieve the ce intended by the urer, i.e., be designed and ured in such a way, that they le for sone or more of the referred to in Article 1(2)(a) as by the manufacturer.	A	Internal Internal	Specification reviews Validation testing		P

Figure 21-1 Sample Essential Requirements list. (From Fries, 1995)

and which has its reference published in the *Official Journal of the European Communities*.

The Essential Requirements are worded such that they identify a risk and state that the device should be designed and manufactured to ensure the risk is avoided or minimized. The technical detail for ensuring these requirements is to be found in Harmonized Standards. Manufacturers must therefore identify the Harmonized Standards corresponding to the Essential Requirements which apply to their device.

With regard to choosing such standards, the manufacturer must be aware of the hierarchy of standards which have been developed:

- Horizontal Standards: Generic standards covering fundamental requirements common to all, or a very wide range of medical devices.
- Semi-Horizontal Standards: Group standards which deal with requirements applicable to a group of devices.
- Vertical Standards: Product-specific standards which give requirements to one device or a very small group of devices.

Manufacturers must give particular attention to the horizontal standards since, because of their general nature, they apply to almost all devices. As these standards come into use for almost all products, they will become extremely powerful.

Semi-horizontal standards may be particularly important as they have virtually the same weight as horizontal standards for groups of devices, such as orthopedic implants, IVDs, or X-ray equipment.

Vertical standards might well be too narrow to cope with new technological developments when a question of a specific feature of a device arises.

The following are medical standards applicable to the Medical Device Directives.

General Requirements for Safety

Standard	Content
-	
IEC 601-1-1	Collateral standard on safety requirements
IEC 60601-1-2	Collateral standard on electromagnetic compatibility
IEC 60601-1-3	Collateral standard on radiation protection in diagnostic X-ray equipment.

Particular Requirements for Safety

Standard	Content
-	
IEC 601-2-2	High frequency surgical equipment
EN 60601-2-21	Infant radiant warmers
EN 60601-2-22	Diagnostic and therapeutic laser equipment
EN 60601-2-26	Electroencephalographs
EN 60601-2-28	Diagnostic X-ray sources and tube assemblies
EN 60601-2-30	Auto-cycling indirect blood pressure monitors
EN 60601-2-31	External cardiac pacemakers with internal power
EN 60601-2-32	Associated equipment of X-ray equipment
EN 60601-2-34	Direct blood pressure monitoring equipment.

21.2.4 Assurance That the Device Meets the Essential Requirements and Harmonized Standards and Documentation of the Evidence

Once the Essential Requirements List has been developed and the harmonized standards chosen, the activity to prove the Essential Requirements List must be conducted. Taking the activity on the Essential Requirements checklist from Figure 21-1, the following activity may be conducted to ensure the requirements are met.

Essential Requirement 1

This requirement is concerned with the device not compromising the clinical condition or the safety of patient, users, and where applicable, other persons.

The methods used to meet this requirement are the conduction of a hazard analysis and a safety review.

A hazard analysis is the process, continuous throughout the product development cycle, that examines the possible hazards that could occur due to equipment failure and helps the designer to eliminate the hazard through various control methods. The hazard analysis is conducted on hardware, software, and the total system during the initial specification phase and is updated throughout the development cycle. The hazard analysis is documented on a form similar to that shown in Figure 21-2.

The hazard analysis addresses the following issues:

Potential Hazard	Identifies possible harm to patient, operator, or system.
Generic Cause	Identifies general conditions that can lead to the associated Potential Hazard.
Specific Cause	Identifies specific instances that can give rise to the associated Generic Cause.
Probability	Classifies the likelihood of the associated Potential Hazard according to Table 21-1.
Severity	Categorizes the associated Potential Hazard according to Table 21-2.
Control Mode	Means of reducing the probability and/or severity of the associated Potential Hazard.

Control Method	Actual implementation to achieve the associated Control Mode.
Comments	Additional information, references, etc.
Review Comments	Comments written down during the review meeting.

Potential hazard	Generic cause	Specific cause	Probability	Severity	Control mode	Control method	Comments	R con

Figure 21-2 Sample Hazard Analysis form. (From Fries, 1997)

Classification Indicator	Classification Rating	Classification Meaning
1	Frequent	Likely to occur often
2	Occasional	Will occur several times in the life of the device
3	Reasonably Remote	Likely to occur sometime in the life of the device
4	Remote	Unlikely to occur, but possible
5	Extremely Remote	Probability of occurrence indistinguishable from zero
6	Physically Impossible	

Table 21-1 Hazard Analysis Probability Classification (From Fries, 1997)

When the hazard analysis is initially completed, the probability and severity refer to the potential hazard prior to its being controlled. As the device is designed to minimize or eliminate the hazard, and control methods are imposed, the probability and severity will be updated.

An organization separate from R&D, such as Quality Assurance, reviews the device to ensure it is safe and effective for its intended use. The device, when operated according to specification, must not cause a hazard to the user or the patient. In the conduction of this review, the following may be addressed:

- Pertinent documentation such as drawings, test reports, and manuals
- A sample of the device
- A checklist specific to the device, which may include:
    - Voltages
    - Operating frequencies
    - Leakage currents
    - Dielectric withstand
    - Grounding impedance
    - Power cord and plug
    - Electrical insulation
    - Physical stability

Severity Indicator	Severity Rating	Severity Meaning
I	Catastrophic	May cause death or device loss
II	Critical	May cause *severe* injury, occupational illness, or system damage
III	Marginal	May cause *minor* injury, occupational illness, or system damage
IV	Negligible	Will not result in injury, illness, system damage

Table 21-2 Hazard Analysis Severity Classification (From Fries, 1997)

- Color coding
- Circuit breakers and fuses
- Alarms, warnings, and indicators
- Mechanical design integrity.

The checklist is signed by the reviewing personnel following the analysis.

Essential Requirement 2

This requirement is concerned with the device complying with safety principles and the generally acknowledged state of the art. The methods used to meet this requirement are peer reviews and the safety review.

Peer review of the Product Specification, Design Specification, Software Requirements Specification, and the actual design are conducted using qualified individuals not directly involved in the development of the device. The review is attended by individuals from Design, Reliability, Quality Assurance, Regulatory Affairs, Marketing, Manufacturing, and Service departments. Each review is documented with issues discussed and action items. After the review, the project team assigns individuals to address each action item and a schedule for completion.

The safety review was discussed under Essential Requirement 1.

Essential Requirement 3

This requirement is concerned with the device achieving the performance intended by the manufacturer. The methods used to meet this requirement are the various specification reviews and the validation of the device to meet those specifications.

Specification Reviews were discussed under Essential Requirement 2.

Validation Testing involves ensuring that the design and the product meet the appropriate specifications that were developed at the beginning of the development process. Testing is conducted to address each requirement in the specification and the test plan and test results documented. It is helpful to develop a requirements matrix to assist in this activity.

Essential Requirement 4

This requirement is concerned with the device being adversely affected by stresses which can occur during normal conditions of use. The methods used to meet this requirement are environmental testing, Environmental Stress Screening (ESS), and use/misuse evaluation.

Environmental testing is conducted according to Environmental Specifications listed for the product. Table 21-3 lists the environmental testing to be conducted and the corresponding standards and methods employed.

Test results are documented.

During Environmental Stress Screening (ESS) the device is subjected to temperature and vibration stresses beyond that which the device may ordinarily see in order to precipitate failures. The failure may then be designed out of the device before it is produced. ESS is conducted according to a specific protocol which is developed for the particular device. Care must be taken in preparing the protocol to avoid causing failures which would not ordinarily be anticipated. Results of the ESS analysis are documented.

Whether through failure to properly read the operation manual or through improper training, medical devices are going to be misused and even abused. There are many stories of product misuse, such as the hand-held monitor that was dropped into a toilet bowl, the physician that hammered a 9-volt battery in backwards and then reported the device was not working, or the user that spilled a can of soda on and into a device.

Environmental Test	Specification Range	Applicable Standard
Operating Temperature	5° to 35°C	IEC 68-2-14
Storage Temperature	-40° to +65°C	IEC 68-2-1-Ab IEC 68-2-2-Bb
Operating Humidity	15 to 95% RH non-condensing	IEC 68-2-30
Operating Pressure	500 to 797 mm Hg	IEC 68-2-13
Storage Pressure	87 to 797 mm Hg	IEC 68-2-13
Radiated Electrical Emissions	4 dB margin	CISPR 11
Radiated Magnetic Emissions	4 dB margin	VDE 871
Line Conducted Emissions	2 dB margin	CISPR 11 VDE 871
Electrostatic Discharge	Contact: 7KV Air: 10 KV	EN 60601-2 EN 1000-4-2
Radiated Electric Field Immunity	5 V/m @ 1KHz	EN 60601-2 EN 1000-4-3
Electrical Fast Transient Immunity	Mains: 2.4 KV Cables >3m: 1.2 KV	EN 60601-2 EN 1000-4-4
Stability		UL 2601
Transportation		NSTA

Table 21-3 Sample of Environmental Testing (From Fries, 1997.)

Practically, it is impossible to make a device completely misuse-proof, but it is highly desirable to design around the misuse situations than can be anticipated. These include:

- Excess application of cleaning solutions
- Physical abuse

- Spills
- Excess weight applied to certain parts of the device
- Excess torque applied to controls or screws
- Improper voltages, frequencies, or pressures
- Interchangeable electrical or pneumatic connections.

Each potential misuse situation should be evaluated for its possible result on the device and a decision made on whether the result can be designed out.

Activities similar to these are carried out to complete the remainder of the Essential Requirements checklist for the device.

21.2.5 Classification of the Device

It is necessary for the manufacturer of a medical device to have some degree of proof that a device complies with the Essential Requirements before the CE marking can be applied. This is defined as a "conformity assessment procedure." For devices applicable to the AIMDD, there two alternatives for the conformity assessment procedure. For devices applicable to the IVDMDD, there is a single conformity assessment procedure. For devices applicable to the MDD, there is no conformity assessment procedure that is suitable for all products, as the directive covers all medical devices. Medical devices are therefore divided into four classes, which have specific conformity assessment procedures for each of the four classes.

The key to the classification process is a clear understanding of the intended purpose of the device. If the device is used for more than one intended purpose, then it must be classified according to the one which gives the highest classification. The Classification Rules are found in Annex IX of the Medical Device Directive.

21.2.6 Decision on the Appropriate Conformity Assessment Procedure

<u>Medical Devices Directive</u>

There are six conformity assessment Annexes to the Medical Devices Directive. Their use for the different classes of devices is specified in Article 11 of the Directive.

- Annex II: This Annex describes the system of full quality assurance covering both the design and manufacture of devices.

- Annex III: This Annex describes the type of examination procedure according to which the manufacturer submits full technical documentation of the product, together with a representative sample of the device to a Notified Body.

- Annex IV: Under this procedure, the Notified Body examines every individual product, or one or more samples from every production batch and carries out such tests as are necessary to show the conformity of the products with the approved/documented design.

- Annex V: This Annex describes a production quality system which is to be verified by a Notified Body as ensuring that devices are made in accordance with an approved type, or in accordance with technical documentation describing the device.

- Annex VI: This Annex describes a quality system covering final inspection and testing of products to ensure that devices are made in accordance with an approved type, or in accordance with technical documentation.

- Annex VII: This Annex describes the technical documentation that the manufacturer must compile in order to support a declaration of conformity for a medical device, where there is no participation of a Notified Body in the process.

The class to which the medical device is assigned has an influence on the type of conformity assessment procedure chosen.

- Class I: Compliance with the Essential Requirements must be shown in technical documentation compiled according to Annex VII of the Directive.

- Class IIa: The design of the device and it compliance with the Essential Requirements must be established in technical documentation described in Annex VII.

agreement of production units with the technical documentation must be ensured by a Notified Body according to one of the following alternatives:

- sample testing: Annex IV
- an audited production quality system: Annex V
- an audited product quality system: Annex VI

- Class IIb: The design and manufacturing procedures must be approved by a Notified Body as satisfying Annex II, or the design must be shown to conform to the Essential Requirements by a type examination (Annex III) carried out by a Notified Body.

- Class III: The procedures for this class are similar to Class IIb, but significant differences are that when the quality system route is used, a design dossier for each type of device must be examined by the Notified Body. Clinical data relating to safety and performance must be included in the design dossier or the documentation presented for the type examination.

Active Implantable Medical Devices Directive

For devices following the AIMDD, Annexes II through V cover the various conformity assessment procedures available. There are two alternative procedures:

Alternative 1

A manufacturer must have in place a full Quality Assurance system for design and production and must submit a design dossier on each type of device to the Notified Body for review.

Alternative 2

A manufacturer submits an example of each type of device to a Notified Body. Satisfactory production must be achieved by ensuring either the quality system at the manufacturing site complies with EN 29002 and EN 46002 and has been audited by a Notified Body, or samples of the product must be tested by a Notified Body.

In Vitro Diagnostic Medical Devices Directive

For devices adhering to the IVDMDD, the conformity assessment procedure is a manufacturer's declaration. In vitro devices for self testing, additionally must have a design examination by a Notified Body, or be designed and manufactured in accordance with a quality system.

In choosing a conformity assessment procedure it is important to remember that 1) it is essential to determine the classification of a device before deciding on a conformity assessment procedure, 2) it may be more efficient to operate one conformity assessment procedure throughout a manufacturing plant, even though this procedure may be more rigorous than strictly necessary for some products, and 3) tests and assessments carried out under current national regulations can contribute toward the assessment of conformity with the requirements of the directives.

21.2.7 Identification and Choice of a Notified Body

Identifying and choosing a Notified Body is one of the most critical issues facing a manufacturer. A long-term and close relationship should be developed and time and care spent in making a careful choice of a Notified Body should be viewed as an investment in the future of the company.

Notified Bodies must satisfy the criteria given in Annex XI of the Medical Devices Directive, namely:

- independence from the design, manufacture, or supply of the devices in question
- integrity
- competence
- staff who are trained, experienced, and able to report
- impartiality of the staff
- possession of liability insurance
- professional secrecy.

In addition, the bodies must satisfy the criteria fixed by the relevant Harmonized Standards. The relevant Harmonized Standards include those of the EN 45000 series dealing with the accreditation and operation of certification bodies.

The tasks to be carried out by Notified Bodies include:

- audit manufacturers; quality systems for compliance with Annexes II, V, and VI
- examine any modifications to an approved quality system
- carry out periodic surveillance of approved quality systems
- examine design dossiers and issue EC Design Examination Certificates
- examine modifications to an approved design
- carry out type examinations and issue EC Type Examination Certificates
- examine modifications to an approved type
- carry out EC verification
- take measures to prevent rejected batches from reaching the market
- agree with the manufacturer time limits for the conformity assessment procedures
- take into account the results of tests or verifications already carried out
- communicate to other Notified Bodies (on request) all relevant information about approvals of quality systems issued, refused, and withdrawn
- communicate to other Notified Bodies (on request) all relevant information about EC Type Approval Certificates issued, refused, and withdrawn.

Notified bodies must be located within the European Community in order that effective control may be applied by the Competent Authorities that appointed them, but certain operations may be carried out on behalf of Notified Bodies by subcontractors who may be based outside the European Community. Competent Authorities will generally notify bodies on their own territory, but they may notify bodies based in another Member State provided that they have already been notified by their parent Competent Authority.

There are several factors to be taken into account by a manufacturer in choosing a Notified Body, including:

- experience with medical devices
- range of medical devices for which the Notified Body has skills

- possession of specific skills, e.g., EMC or software
- links with subcontractors and subcontractor skills
- conformity assessment procedures for which the body is notified
- plans for handling issues, such as clinical evaluation
- attitude to existing certifications
- queue times/processing times
- costs
- location and working languages.

Experience with medical devices is limited to a small number of test houses and their experience is largely confined to electromedical equipment. Manufacturers should probe carefully the competence of the certification body to assess their device. Actual experience with a product of a similar nature would be reensuring. The certification body should be pressed to demonstrate sufficient understanding of the requirements, particularly where special processes are involved (e.g., sterilization) and/or previous experience.

Certain devices demand specific skills which may not be found in every Notified Body. Clearly, the Notified Body must have, or be able to obtain, the skills required for the manufacturer's devices.

Many Notified Bodies will supplement their in-house skills by the use of specialist subcontractors. This is perfectly acceptable as long as all the rules of subcontracting are followed. Manufacturers should verify for themselves the reputation of the subcontractor and the degree of supervision applied by the Notified Body.

The main choice open to manufacturers is full Quality System certification or Type Examination combined with one of the less rigorous Quality System certifications. Some Notified Bodies have a tradition of either product testing or systems evaluation and it therefore makes sense to select a Notified Body with experience in the route chosen.

A clinical evaluation is required for some medical devices, especially Class III devices and implants. Although this will be a key aspect of demonstrating conformity, it will be important for manufacturers to know how the Notified Body intends to perform this function.

In preparing the Medical Devices Directives, the need to avoid re-inventing the wheel has been recognized. In order to maximize this need, companies whose products have already been certified by test houses which are likely to become Notified Bodies may wish to make use of the organizations with whom they have previously worked. It will be important to verify with the Notified Body the extent to which the testing previously performed is sufficient to meeting the Essential Requirements.

At the time of this writing, most Notified Bodies seem to be able to offer fairly short lead times. The time for actually carrying out the examination or audit should be questioned.

It must be remembered that manufacturers will have to pay Notified Bodies for carrying out the conformity assessment procedures. There will certainly be competition and this may offer some control over costs. Although it will always be a factor, the choice of a Notified Body should not be governed by cost alone bearing in mind the importance of the exercise.

For obvious reasons of expense, culture, convenience and language there will be a tendency for European manufacturers to use a Notified Body situated in their own country. Nevertheless, this should not be the principal reason for selection and account should be taken of the other criteria discussed here. For manufacturers outside the European Community, the geographical locations is less important. Of greater significance to them, particularly U.S. companies, is the existence of overseas subsidiaries or subcontractors of some of the Notified Bodies. Manufacturers should understand that the Notified Body must be a legal entity established within the Member State which has notified it. This does not prevent the Notified Body subcontracting quite significant tasks to a subsidiary.

Article 11.12 states that the correspondence relating to the conformity assessment procedures must be in the language of the Member State in which the procedures are carried out and/or in another European Community language acceptable to the Notified Body. Language may thus be another factor affecting the choice of Notified Body, although most of the major certification bodies will accept English and other languages.

The most significant factor of all is likely to be existing good relations with a particular body. Notified Bodies will be drawn from existing test and certification bodies and many manufacturers already use such bodies, either as part of a national approval procedure, or as part of their own policy for ensuring the satisfactory quality of their products and processes.

Another consideration which could become significant is that of variations in the national laws implementing the directives. Notified Bodies will have to apply the law of the country in which they are situated and some differences in operation could be introduced by this means.

21.2.8 Obtaining Conformity Certifications

Certificates of conformity will be given by the establishment conducting the test. A copy of the test report, including all test results, should accompany the certificates and be placed in the Technical File.

21.2.9 Establishing a Declaration of Conformity

Of all documents prepared for the Medical Devices Directives, the most important may be the declaration of conformity. Every device, other than a custom-made or clinical investigation device, must be covered by a declaration of conformity.

The general requirement is that the manufacturer shall draw up a written declaration that the products concerned meet the provisions of the directive that apply to them. The declaration must cover a given number of the products manufactured. A strictly literal interpretation of this wording would suggest that the preparation of a declaration of conformity is not a one-and-for-all event with an indefinite coverage, but rather a formal statement that products which have been manufactured and verified in accordance with the particular conformity assessment procedure chosen by the manufacturer do meet the requirements of the directive. Such an interpretation would impose severe burdens on manufacturers, and the Commission is understood to be moving to a position where a declaration of conformity can be prepared in respect of future production of a model of device for which the conformity assessment procedures have been carried out. The CE marking of individual devices after manufacture can then be regarded as a short-form expression of the declaration of conformity in respect of that individual device. This position is likely to form part of future Commission guidance.

Even so, the declaration remains a very formal statement from the manufacturer and accordingly, must be drawn up with care. The declaration must include the serial numbers or batch numbers of the products it covers and manufacturers should give careful thought to the appropriate coverage of a declaration. In the extreme, it may be that a separate declaration should be prepared individually for each product or batch.

A practical approach is probably to draw up one basic declaration which is stated to apply to the products whose serial (batch) numbers are listed in an Appendix. The Appendix can then be ammended to at sensible intervals.

A suggested format for the Declaration of Conformity is shown in Figure 21-3.

21.2.10 Application of the CE Mark

The CE marking (Figure 21-4) is the symbol used to indicate that a particular product complies with the relevant Essential Requirements of the appropriate directive, and as such, that the product has achieved a satisfactory level of safety and thus may circulate freely throughout the European Community.

It is important to note that it is the manufacturer or their authorized representative who applies the CE marking to the product, and not the Notified Body. The responsibility for ensuring that each and every product conforms to the requirements of the directive is that of the manufacturer and the affixing of the CE marking constitutes the manufacturer's statement that an individual device conforms.

The CE marking should appear on the device itself, if practicable, on the instructions for use, and on the shipping packaging. It should be accompanied by the identification number of the Notified Body which has been involved in the verification of the production of the device. It is prohibited to add other marks which could confuse or obscure the meaning of the CE marking.

The XXXX noted in Figure 21-4 is the identification number of the notified body.

We: Company Name
Company Address

Declare that the product(s) listed below:

Product to be declared

Hereby conform(s) to the European Council Directive 93/42/EEC, Medical Device Directive, Annex II, Article 3. This declaration is based on the Certification of the Full Quality Assurance System by NAME OF NOTIFIED BODY, Notified Body # XXXX.

Name (*Print or type*) : ____________________
Title : ____________________
Signature : ____________________
Date : ____________________

Figure 21-3 Sample Declaration of Conformity. (From Fries, 1997)

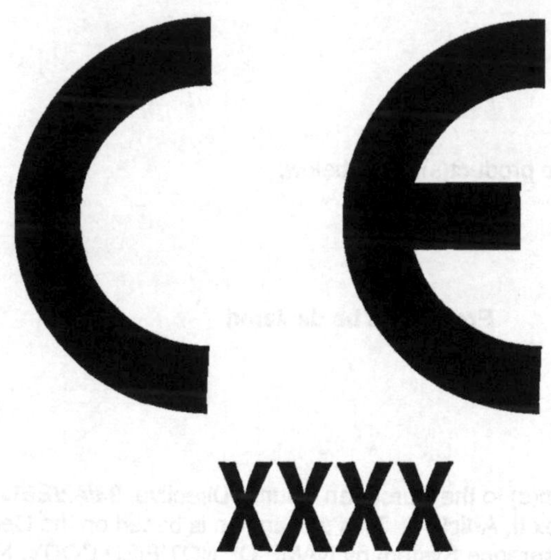

Figure 21-4 Example of CE Mark. (From Fries, 1997)

References

The Active Implantable Medical Devices Directive. 90/385/EEC, 20 June, 1990.

The Medical Devices Directive. 93/42/EEC, 14 June, 1993.

Draft Proposal for a Council Directive on In Vitro Diagnostic Medical Devices, Working Document. III/D/4181/93, April, 1993.

Fries, R.C. and M. Graber, "Designing Medical Devices for Conformance with Harmonized Standards," *Biomedical Instrumentation & Technology.* Volume 29, Number 4, July/August, 1995.

Fries, Richard C., *Reliable Design of Medical Devices.* New York: Marcel Dekker, Inc., 1997.

Higson, G.R., *The Medical Devices Directive-A Manufacturer's Handbook.* Brussels: Medical Technology Consultants Europe Ltd., 1993.

SWBC, Organization for the European Conformity of Products, *CE-Mark: The New European Legislation for Products.* Milwaukee, WI: ASQC Quality Press, 1996.

Chapter 22

Quality System Regulations

Nearly twenty years ago, the United States Food and Drug Administration established its Good Manufacturing Practices (GMP) for both domestic and foreign manufacturers of medical devices intended for human use. The agency took the position that the failure of manufacturers to follow good manufacturing practices was responsible for a substantial number of device failures and recalls.

The philosophy behind the FDA's requirement that manufacturers adopt GMPs is simple. While the agency's premarket review of devices serves as a check of their safety and effectiveness, it was felt that only compliance with GMPs could ensure that devices were produced in a reliable and consistent manner. At that time, the original GMPs did not in themselves guarantee that a product that was once shown to be safe and effective could be reliably produced.

Recently, spurred by an act of Congress, the FDA has changed its regulations, adding a requirement for design controls and bringing U.S. GMPs into substantive harmony with international requirements. The addition of design controls changes the very nature of the GMP requirements, which now seek to increase the chances that devices will be designed in such a manner as to be safe, effective, and reliable. Further, with the agency embracing the goal of international harmonization, the day may not be far off when manufacturers will be able to establish a single set of manufacturing practices that will satisfy regulatory requirements from New Zealand to Norway. Indeed, the agency has already spoken publicly about the mutual recognition of inspection results among industrialized countries, and has even raised the possibility of third-party audits to replace the need for some FDA inspections.

22.1 History of the Quality System Regulations

Like most U.S. medical device law, the Current Good Manufacturing Practices requirements trace their genesis to the medical device amendments of 1976. Section 520(f) of the Federal Food, Drug, and Cosmetic Act authorized the FDA to establish GMPs. On July 21, 1978, the agency issued its original GMP regulations, which described the facilities and methods to be used in the manufacture, packaging, storage, and installation of medical devices. Aside from some editorial comments, these requirements would remain unchanged for nearly 20 years.

In 1990, Congress passed the Safe Medical Device Act, which gave the FDA authority to add "preproduction design validation controls" to the GMP regulations. The act also encouraged the FDA to work with foreign countries toward mutual recognition of GMP inspections.

The agency went right to work on this and in June, 1990 proposed revised GMPs. Almost seven years of debate and revision followed, but finally, on October 7, 1996, the FDA issued its final rules. The new Quality System Regulations, incorporating the required design controls, went into effect June 1, 1997. The design control provisions, however, will not be enforced until June 14, 1998.

The design controls embodied in the new regulations were necessary, the FDA stated, because the lack of such controls had been a major cause of device recalls in the past. A 1990 study suggested that approximately 44% of the quality problems that had led to voluntary recall actions in the previous six years were attributable to errors or deficiencies designed into particular devices, deficiencies that might have been prevented had design controls been in place. With respect to design flaws in software, the data were even more alarming: one study of software related recalls indicated that more than 90% were due to design errors.

Like their predecessors, the new rules are broadly stated. "Because this regulation must apply to so many different types of devices, the regulation does not prescribe in detail how a manufacturer must produce a specific device," explained the FDA. The rules apply to all Class II and Class III devices and to some Class I devices. Failure to comply with the provisions will automatically render any device produced "adulterated" and subject to FDA sanction.

22.2 Scope

On October 7, 1996, FDA published the long-awaited revision of its medical device good manufacturing practices (GMP) regulation in the Federal Register. Manufacturers that have not remained current with the changes in the regulation that the agency has proposed over the past six years are in for a major surprise. And even those that have kept current with the agency's proposals up through the working draft of July 1995 will find a few new twists.

Now renamed as a quality system regulation, FDA's new revision differs significantly from the previous GMP regulation of 1978. It also adds a number of requirements not present in the agency's proposed rule of November 1993, and introduces a number of changes developed since publication of the July 1995 working draft. Specifically, the new quality system regulation contains major additional requirements in the areas of design, management responsibility, purchasing, and servicing.

It is clear that the new regulation has been greatly influenced by the work of the Global Harmonization Task Force. In slightly different wording, the regulation now incorporates all the requirements of the fullest of the quality systems standards compiled by the International Organization for Standardization (ISO). For example, there are now requirements for quality planning, for a quality manual, and for an outline of the general quality procedure. All these new requirements were added in order to bring the regulation into harmony with the quality systems standards currently accepted in the member nations of the European Union (EU), and there is certainly a benefit to their inclusion in the new regulation.

But the regulation also adds documentation requirements that would not have been included if harmonization were not an agency goal, and these requirements must now be met by all U.S. device manufacturers--even if they do not intend to export to the EU. On the up side, the language of the new regulation will allow manufacturers much more flexibility than either the November 1993 proposal or July 1995 working draft would have allowed.

Section 22.3 will review the changes that the agency has incorporated into the sections of its newest regulation and will discuss how those changes are likely to affect device manufacturers.

22.3 General Provisions

As mentioned above, FDA has changed the title of its revised regulation from "Good Manufacturing Practice for Medical Devices" to "Quality System Regulation." This change is more than just a matter of nomenclature; it is intended to reflect the expanded scope of the new regulation as well as to bring its terminology into harmony with that of the ISO 9000 family of quality systems standards. While the 1978 GMP regulation focused almost exclusively on production practices, the new regulation encompasses quality system requirements that apply to the entire life cycle of a device. The new rule is therefore properly referred to as a quality system regulation, into which the agency's revised requirements for good manufacturing practices have been incorporated.

The 1978 GMP regulation was a two-tier regulation that included general requirements applicable to all devices and additional requirements that applied only to critical ones. In the new quality system regulation, the notion of a critical device has been removed, and the term is no longer used. However, the new regulation's section on traceability (820.65) makes use of the same general concept, and the definition of traceable device found there is the same as the definition of critical device as presented in the 1978 GMP regulation (820.3(f)). Other critical-device requirements of the 1978 GMP regulation have been melded into appropriate sections of the quality system regulation; for instance, the critical operation requirements are now included in the section on process validation (820.75).

The new regulation's section on scope makes it clear that manufacturers need only comply with those parts of the regulation that apply to them. Thus, for example, only manufacturers who service devices need comply with the servicing requirements. Like the 1978 GMP regulation, the quality system regulation does not apply to component manufacturers, but they are encouraged to use it for guidance.

One important statement in the new regulation's section on scope is the definition of the phrase "where appropriate," which is used in reference to a number of requirements. Contrary to what manufacturers might hope, this phrase doesn't limit application of the regulation's requirements to times when manufacturers believe they are appropriate. Instead, FDA means that a requirement should be considered appropriate "if nonimplementation could reasonably be expected to result in the product not meeting its specified requirements or the manufacturer not being able to carry out any necessary corrective action." In short, a requirement is considered appropriate unless the manufacturer can document justification to the contrary. Unfortunately, industry was not provided an opportunity to comment on the agency's use of this phrase.

Another important issue covered under the scope of the new regulation relates to foreign firms that export devices to the United States. The agency has routinely inspected such firms to determine whether they are complying with GMPs although it has no authority to do so, and must rely on an invitation from the company in question. Some foreign manufacturers have refused to allow FDA to inspect their facilities. The new regulation's section on scope addresses this situation by stating that devices produced by foreign manufacturers that refuse to permit FDA inspections will be considered adulterated and will be detained by U.S. Customs. FDA is basing its authority to impose this penalty on the Federal Food, Drug, and Cosmetic Act (Section 801(a)). It will be interesting to see what occurs if a foreign manufacturer chooses to challenge this position.

References

Dash, Glenn, "CGMPs for Medical Device Manufacturers," in *Compliance Engineering.* Volume 14, Number 2, March-April, 1997.

European Committee for Standardization, "Quality Systems--Medical Devices--Particular Requirements for the Application of EN 29001," *European Norm 46001*, Brussels, European Committee for Standardization, 1996.

Food and Drug Administration, "Medical Devices; Current Good Manufacturing Practice (CGMP) Final Rule; Quality System Regulation," *Federal Register.* October 7, 1996.

Food and Drug Administration, Code of Federal Regulations, 21 CFR 820, "Good Manufacturing Practice for Medical Devices," *Federal Register.* July 21, 1978.

Food and Drug Administration, "Medical Devices; Current Good Manufacturing Practice (CGMP) Regulations; Proposed Revisions; Request for Comments," *Federal Register*. November 23, 1993.

Food and Drug Administration, "Medical Devices; Working Draft of the Current Good Manufacturing Practice (CGMP) Final Rule; Notice of Availability; Request for Comments; Public Meeting," *Federal Register*. July 24, 1995.

Global Harmonization Task Force, "Guidance on Quality Systems for the Design and Manufacture of Medical Devices," Issue 7, August 1994.

International Organization for Standardization, "Quality Systems--Model for Quality Assurance in Design, Development, Production, Installation, and Servicing," *ISO 9001:1994*, Geneva: International Organization for Standardization (ISO), 1994.

Chapter 23

Quality System Regulation Requirements and Compliance

The Quality System Regulations (revised GMP) were issued on October 7, 1996. The Quality System Regulations, incorporating design controls, went into effect June 1, 1997, though the design-control provision will not be enforced until June 1, 1998. Like its predecessors, the new regulations are broadly stated, because the regulations must apply to many different types of devices. Failure to comply with the provisions will automatically render any device produced *adulterated* and subject to FDA sanction.

One of the FDA's goals is to harmonize its Quality System Regulation requirements with the international standard ISO 9001:1994 and with the ISO standard ISO/DIS 13485. This is all part of a broader effort to foster international harmonization of standards and mutual recognition of inspections, work that is being undertaken largely by the Global Harmonization Task Force.

23.1 Quality System

23.1.1 Regulation

Each manufacturer must establish and maintain a quality system that is appropriate for the specific medical devices designed or manufactured.

23.1.2 Compliance

The regulations make it clear that it is the responsibility of executive management to establish a quality system and to ensure that it is both implemented and understood at all levels of the organization. A member of management must be appointed whose assigned role is to ensure that the quality system requirements are effectively established and maintained, and to report to management on the system. The use of the term *establish* indicates that the requirements must be documented, either in writing or electronically, and then implemented.

Management will need to establish a procedure for auditing the quality system. The requirements provide that quality audits must be conducted by individuals who do not have direct responsibility for the area being audited. Corrective actions, including a re-audit of deficient matters, must be taken when necessary. Although the frequency of the audits is not specified, it should be determined by the organization and documented.

Manufacturers must have sufficient personnel and must establish procedures by which they may identify training needs. Training must be documented. All personnel, not just those involved in the quality system, must be made aware of the device defects that could result from the improper performance of their job. Those involved with verification and validation activities must additionally be familiarized with the particular defects and errors they may encounter.

All personnel must have the necessary background, education, and training to perform their tasks. Formal training programs are not always required. For most operations, on-the-job training is sufficient. The agency is likely, however, to require formal training for persons involved in those areas that may be especially prone to problems.

23.2 Design Controls

23.2.1 Requirements

Each manufacturer of any Class II or Class III device, and the Class I devices listed in the regulations, must establish and maintain procedures to control the design of the device in order to ensure that specified design requirements are met.

Each manufacturer must establish and maintain plans that describe or reference the design and development activities and define responsibility.

Each manufacturer must establish and maintain procedures to ensure that design requirements address the intended use of the device, including the needs of the user and the patient.

Each manufacturer must establish and maintain procedures for definin and documenting design output in terms that allow an adequate evaluation of conformance to design input requirements. Design output procedures must contain or make reference to acceptance criteria.

Each manufacturer must establish and maintain procedures to ensure that formal documented reviews of the design results are planned and conducte at appropriate stages.

Design verification must confirm that the design output meets the design input requirements.

Design validation must be performed under defined operating conditions on initial production units. Design validation must ensure that devices conform to defined user needs and intended uses and must include testing of production units under actual or simulated use conditions.

Each manufacturer must establish and maintain procedures to ensure that the device is correctly translated into production specifications.

Each manufacturer must establish and maintain procedures for the identification, documentation, validation, or where appropriate, verification, review, and approval of design changes.

23.2.2 Compliance

Records demonstrating that the device has been developed in accordance with these requirements must be kept in a Design History File (DHF). The Design History File is defined as:

> a compilation of records that describes
> the design history of a finished device.

It should be distinguished from other, similarly named records required elsewhere in the regulations, such as the Device Master Record and the Device History Record.

The Design and Development Plan serves as a road map for the development process. It describes the kinds of activities that are to be undertaken and identifies who is responsible for each. Once of these activities will be the establishment of design inputs, which will require interfacing with other groups, including users and patients. Such interfaces must be documented and the entire plan updated and approved as the design and development evolve. The FDA expects the Design and Development Plan to be explicit enough that employees can determine how inputs are to be gathered, what they are to do, and who is to be responsible for oversight, yet not so detailed as to dictate, for example, what kinds of tools must be used.

Design and Development Plans need not be established when an organization is purely in the research phase of a project, and development is still uncertain. However, once a company has decided to go forward with the product, a Design and Development Plan must be drawn up.

By requiring manufacturers to control the mechanism by which they obtain input for designs, the FDA is requiring that there be an established procedure for identifying precisely how design input is obtained and documented.

The result of the design effort will be the design output, consisting of the design itself, its packaging, labeling, and the Device Master Record, which includes the specifications for the device and the procedures used to build, verify, and validate it. Design output must be documented and approved with the approval bearing the date and signature of the individual responsible.

Design reviews must be performed at appropriate stages in the development process. Present at such reviews should be representatives familiar with each function involved, as well as an individual who does not have direct responsibility for the design stage being reviewed. The FDA has indicated that persons involved in one aspect of a design may serve as independent reviewers for other aspects that they are not involved in, thereby satisfying the independence requirement in even the smallest of companies. The FDA also recommends that functions far removed from the actual design process be represented. The results of the design review, annotated with the date and a list of the individuals present and their titles, must be included in the Design History File.

Design verification and validation are two different things. Verification can be thought of as the measurement of a physical parameter. Validation, by contrast, is a more complex procedure in which a total assessment of the product is undertaken to determine whether it satisfies its intended use, including the needs of users and patients. Verification is a check against an organization's internal standards. Validation reaches out to the product's consumers.

In defining design validation, the international standards upon which the new regulations are based refer to the need to perform clinical evaluations. The similarity of this term to the term "clinical trials" at first raised some alarm, but the FDA has assured the industry that clinical trials need not necessarily be part of design validation. Validation can be performed using historical data, data extracted from literature, or an evaluation of the product conducted by the company's own staff of registered nurses and doctors. An external check through an investigational-device exemption may also be used to validate a product. All of these make up what is referred to as the clinical evaluation.

When all this activity has been completed, the finished product is ready to be transferred from design and development to manufacturing. Written procedures are required that address this transfer. Written procedures are likewise required for the approval, validation, and verification of design changes.

23.3 Document Controls

23.3.1 Requirements

Each manufacturer must establish and maintain procedures to control all documents.

Each manufacturer must designate an individual(s) to review all documents for adequacy and approval, prior to their issuance.

Documents must be available at all locations.

All obsolete documents must be promptly removed.

Changes to documents must be reviewed and approved. Approved changes must be communicated to the appropriate personnel in a timely manner.

23.3.2 Compliance

The FDA views document control as a critical element in maintaining the quality of a product. All change records must include a description of the change, identification of all affected documents, signature of all approving individuals, date of approval, and date when the change became or will become effective. Increasingly, document control is being facilitated electronically. The FDA has proposed a regulation defining the kind of electronic signature to be used (59 FR 45160). This document is to be used only as guidance until the agency make a final determination.

Changes must be approved by an individual serving in the same function as the one who performed the original review and approval, to ensure that the original approver will have the opportunity to review the change. Where such an arrangement is not possible, another individual may be designated, provided that the designation is documented.

23.4 Purchasing Controls

23.4.1 Requirements

Each manufacturer must establish and maintain procedures to ensure that all purchased or otherwise received product and services conform to specified requirements.

Each manufacturer must establish and maintain the requirements that must be met by suppliers, contractors, and consultants. Each manufacturer must 1) evaluate and select on the basis of their ability to meet the specified requirements, 2) define the type and extent of control to be exercised, and 3) establish and maintain records of acceptable suppliers, contractors, and consultants.

Each manufacturer must establish and maintain data that clearly describe or reference the specified requirements for purchased or otherwise received product and services.

23.4.2 Compliance

Components that are incorporated into finished devices and materials that are used in their manufacture, must also be properly tested or inspected to determine that they meet documented standards. They must then be identified in such a way as to ensure that only acceptable components or materials will be used in manufacturing.

Well-known, industry-standard components may need only a minimum of testing and inspection, while newer and critical components will require more detailed examination. In either case, a record of qualification should be maintained, specifying the component's identity, the particular test/inspection method used, and the result obtained. Component specifications may include dimensions, materials, viscosity, and other features, though for routine standard components, a catalog description may be enough. Quality levels should also be noted, especially for components that are available in several variants, such as industrial, reagent, or military grade.

All components will need to undergo at least a visual inspection. As for testing, it is left to the manufacturer's discretion to decide which components should be individually tested and which should be sampled. In general, some form of testing should be performed if deviations could cause the product to be unfit for its intended use. Manufacturers that decided not to sample or test components should be prepared to justify their decisions, whether on the basis of the supplier's previous performance, a component's known performance history, its application, or other criteria.

Rejected, obsolete, or deteriorated components should be placed in a separate, quarantined area. Records should be kept to document their disposition, stating whether the components were returned or scrapped. In smaller firms, the disposition can be noted directly on the purchase order.

Those components that are accepted should also have their own quarantine area. Components that are liable to be affected by moisture, dirt, or insects should be protected, and those that might degrade should be stored in such a way as to facilitate first-in, first-out (FIFO) use.

Suppliers, consultants, and contractors must also meet specified requirements that should be stated or referenced in the Device Master Record. All evaluations should be documented.

Purchasing documents must include, whenever possible, an agreement that the supplier, contractor, and consultant will notify the manufacturer of any changes so that it may be determined whether or not these will affect the quality of the finished product.

All purchasing data are subject to the document controls outlined in that section.

23.5 Identification and Traceability

23.5.1 Requirements

Each manufacturer must establish and maintain procedures for identifying product during all stages of receipt, production, distribution, and installation to prevent mix-ups.

Each manufacturer of a device that is intended for surgical implant or to support or sustain life and whose failure can be reasonably expected to result in significant injury to the user must establish and maintain procedures for identifying with a control number each unit, lot, or batch.

23.5.2 Compliance

The purpose of the first requirement is to ensure that all products, including components and manufacturing materials, are properly identified so as to prevent mix-ups. The traceability provision applies to the kinds of devices categorized as critical devices in earlier GMPs.

Traceability as referred to in this section is held to apply from the manufacturing facility to the initial consignee. It should be distinguished from FDA tracking requirements, which are used to trace a product all the way to the patient. The tracing of critical components should make up part of the Device History Record.

23.6 Production and Process Controls

23.6.1 Requirements

Each manufacturer must develop, conduct, control, and monitor production processes. Where deviation from device specifications could occur as a result of the manufacturing process, the manufacturer must establish and maintain process control procedures. Process controls must include:

- documented instructions
- monitoring and control of process parameters and component and device characteristics during production
- compliance to specified reference standards or codes
- the approval of process and process equipment
- criteria for workmanship which must be expressed in documented standards or by means of identified and approved representative samples.

Changes must be verified, or where appropriate, validated.

Where environmental conditions could reasonably be expected to have an adverse effect, the manufacturer must establish and maintain procedures to adequately control these environmental conditions.

Each manufacturer must establish and maintain requirements for health, cleanliness, personal practices, and clothing of personnel, if contact could reasonably be expected to have an adverse effect.

Each manufacturer must establish and maintain procedures to prevent contamination.

Buildings must be of suitable design.

Each manufacturer must ensure that all equipment is appropriately designed, constructed, placed, and installed.

Each manufacturer must establish and maintain schedules for the adjustment, cleaning, and other maintenance of equipment.

Each manufacturer must conduct periodic inspections of equipment.

Each manufacturer must ensure that any inherent limitations or allowable tolerances are visibly posted or are readily available.

Where a manufacturing material could reasonably be expected to have an adverse effect, each manufacturer must establish and maintain procedures for the use and removal of such manufacturing material.

When computers or automated data processing systems are used as part of production, the manufacturer must validate the computer software.

Each manufacturer must ensure that all inspection, measuring, and test equipment is suitable for its use and is routinely calibrated, inspected, checked, and maintained.

Calibration procedures must include specific directions and limits for accuracy and precision. When accuracy and precision limits are not met, there must be provisions for remedial action. Calibration must be traceable to national or international standards. Calibration dates, the individual performing each calibration, and the next calibration date must be documented. Calibration records must be displayed on or near each piece of equipment, or shall be readily available.

Where the results of a process cannot be fully verified, the process must be validated.

23.6.2 Compliance

No provision of the regulations is more central to the maintenance of quality standards, or more likely to occupy large amount of the manufacturer's time, money, and attention than this one. The basic philosophy is simple: any possible deviation in the manufacturing process that could affect the quality of the final product must be documented, monitored, and controlled.

Most manufacturers find it helpful to establish standard operating procedures to produce the documents required by this section. Changes to the standard operating procedures must be made in accordance with the section on Document Controls.

Provisions relating to buildings, environment, and personnel have been augmented in the FDA's guidance documents. Buildings should contain sufficient space to allow for proper cleaning, maintenance, and other operations, and should be designed with contamination control in mind. Elements such as humidity, temperature, and static electricity, as well as foreign substances such as paint chips, rust, and microorganisms, should be controlled if they are likely to affect the product adversely. Because overcrowded environments are susceptible to mix-ups, facilities should be laid out with designated, discrete areas for receiving, inspection, testing, manufacturing, labeling, packaging, anc record keeping, with different operations delineated by walls or partitions. Where separate labeling operations are undertaken, each should be treated as a distinct operation, and physically isolated from all other labeling operations.

Even such mundane processes as cleaning should be documented. A record of cleanings should be kept and posted in a convenient location. A notation of mark, an initial, or the signature of the person who performed the cleaning should be entered in this log after each cleanup. Bathrooms and dressing areas should be clean and of adequate size. The use of pesticides in a facility should always be carried out with written procedures. If equipment car be affected by particulates caused by smoking, it is recommended that workers who smoke not enter sensitive portions of the facilities for 15 minutes after smoking.

The regulations also require that equipment used in production be periodically inspected in accordance with a written plan. Inspections need to b documented. Manufacturing materials must be removed if they are likely to have an adverse effect. The removal procedures must be documented, along with the fact of the material's removal. Manufacturing materials do not have t(be eradicated completely. They must, however, be eliminated to the extent tha the amount that remains will not adversely affect the device's quality.

Software used to control manufacturing processes must be validated t(the greatest extent possible. This applies even to off-the-shelf software purchased by the manufacturer, for which assurances must be provided that its performance will match expectations.

Those features of a product that cannot be verified must be controlled through process validation. The FDA defines process validation as:

> establishing documented evidence which provides a high degree of assurance that specific processes will consistently produce product meeting its predetermined specifications anc quality characteristics.

Documented evidence is compiled by challenging the process, that is, by varying input parameters to create worst-case conditions. Parameters include not only component specifications, but also air and water quality and equipmer tolerance levels. Changes to the end product are then measured. Whether or not a product is deemed acceptable will depend on its predetermined specifications. In the case of something simple such as tubing, this could mean the internal and external diameters. Other predetermined specifications could include biocompatibility, durability, and tensile strength.

Validation activities, including the date and signature of the individuals approving the validation, need to be documented. Monitoring methods, data obtained, date, and where appropriate, names of the validating individuals must all be provided. All persons involved must be qualified for their tasks. If and when changes are made to the process, revalidation will be required unless the manufacturer can show why it was not needed.

23.7 Acceptance Activities

23.7.1 Requirements

Each manufacturer shall establish and maintain procedures for acceptance activities.

Incoming products must be inspected, tested, or otherwise verified. Acceptance or rejection must be documented.

Procedures must ensure that in-process product is controlled.

Each manufacturer must ensure that each production run, lot, or batch of finished devices meets acceptance criteria. Finished devices must be held in quarantine or otherwise adequately controlled until release.

Finished devices must not be released for distribution until:

- the activities required in the Device Master Record are completed
- the associated data and documentation are reviewed
- the release is authorized by signature of a designated individual
- the authorization is dated.

Acceptance records must include:

- the acceptance activities performed
- the date acceptance activities were performed

- the results
- the signature of the individual(s) conducting the acceptance activities
- where appropriate, equipment used.

These records must be part of the Device History Record.

Each manufacturer must identify, by suitable means, the acceptance status of product. Acceptance status must be maintained throughout manufacturing, packaging, labeling, installation, and servicing of the product.

23.7.2 Compliance

This section of the regulations is specific to the manufacturer's own acceptance program. The criteria for determining what is acceptable are left to the manufacturer's discretion and may depend, in part, on reasonable reliance on the seller's quality control programs. However, the FDA has indicated that i considers it essential for manufacturers to maintain records of the assessments they perform, with clear indications of pass and fail criteria. All nonconforming product must be dealt with in a specific fashion (see next section).

23.8 Nonconforming Product

23.8.1 Regulations

Each manufacturer shall establish and maintain procedures to control product that does not conform to specified requirements. The procedure must address the identification, documentation, evaluation, segregation, and disposition of nonconforming product. The evaluation of nonconformance mus include a determination of the need for an investigation and notification of the persons or organizations responsible.

Disposition of nonconforming product must be documented.

Each manufacturer shall establish and maintain procedures for rework including testing and reevaluation.

23.8.2 Compliance

This section requires four things of a manufacturer. First, it must set up a program to control the disposition of all nonconforming product. Second, it must ensure that the program addresses the identification, documentation, evaluation, segregation, and disposition of nonconforming product. Third, it must provide for investigations, when necessary. Fourth, it must ensure that such investigations are documented. When an investigation is not undertaken, the rationale for the decision must be documented.

23.9 Corrective and Preventive Action

23.9.1 Regulations

Each manufacturer shall establish and maintain procedures for corrective and preventive action that include:

- analyzing processes, quality audit reports, service records, complaints, and any other sources of quality data to identify existing and potential causes of nonconforming product
- use of appropriate statistical methodology
- investigating the cause of the nonconformity
- identifying the actions required
- verifying or validating the corrective and preventive action
- implementing and recording changes in methods and procedures
- ensuring information related to quality problems or nonconforming product is disseminated to those directly responsible
- submitting relevant information for management review.

All activities required in this section and their results must be documented.

23.9.2 Compliance

Field failures, as well as customer complaints relating to the possible failure of a device to meet any of its specifications, must be reviewed, evaluated, and investigated unless a similar investigation has already been performed. A person or unit needs to be formally designated to carry out this task. The FDA defines a complaint as any expression of dissatisfaction regarding the product's identity, quality, durability, reliability, safety, effectiveness, or performance.

The FDA requires that complaint files be reasonably accessible to investigators and readily available at the manufacturing site. Relabelers, importers, and other entities that distribute products under their own name must forward complaints to the actual manufacturer.

Complaints for a particular product should be grouped in such a way as to enable trends to be identified. According to the FDA, if a manufacturer cannot readily identify defect trends, the firm's management is not complying with the intent of the GMP.

In describing the written procedure that must be followed in the investigation of any outright failure of a device or its components to meet performance specifications, the FDA stipulates that such guidelines must specify that the defective device not be destroyed.

Any deaths related to a device, even those attributable to user error, must also be investigated. Although it is obviously not possible for manufacturers to foresee all conceivable types of misuses, once a potential misuse has come to light, the manufacturer should consider taking corrective and preventative action.

Investigation may be called for even where there is not external complaint. The FDA is of the opinion, for example, that changes in yields mandate the need for investigation.

23.10 Labeling and Packaging Controls

23.10.1 Requirements

Each manufacturer shall establish and maintain procedures to control labeling activities.

Labels must be printed and applied so as to remain legible and affixed during customary conditions.

Labeling must not be released for storage or use until a designated individual(s) has examined the labeling. The release, including the date and signature of the individual(s) performing the examination must be documented in the Device History Record.

Each manufacturer must store labeling in a manner that provides proper identification and is designed to prevent mix-ups.

The label and labeling used must be documented in the Device History Record.

Each manufacturer must ensure that containers are designed and constructed to protect the device from alteration or damage during the customary conditions of processing, storage, handling, and distribution.

23.10.2 Compliance

The precise definitions of the various terms are important here. The term labels is defined as those things that appear on the device itself. Labeling refers to virtually everything else, including dispenser carton labels, case labels, package labels, and directions for use.

The content and design of the labels should be specified or referenced in the Device Master Record, with the specifications to include artwork for each label as well as appropriate inspection and control procedures. The artwork should be accompanied by the name of the preparer, an approval signature, and the approval date. Labels on printed packaging should be treated as components. As such, purchase specifications should define label dimensions, ink, and finish to help ensure that the label and labeling will remain legible throughout the life of the product.

Labels and labeling that have been accepted from vendors should be stored in segregated areas and a documented procedure should be followed when they are released for use. This procedure will need to include a check for any lot numbers or expiration dates. Inspection of the label should be documented on a form that provides the name of the person performing the inspection and its date. Further, since labeling is to be included in the Device Master Record, all changes therein should be performed under the document change control system. Automated label readers, backed up by human oversight, may be used to inspect labels.

Packaging, too, must be evaluated for suitability with special attention paid to devices that must remain sterile, for which some form of validation is usually required. Where products are labeled *sterile* but have not yet been sterilized, a high level of control is required and specific FDA regulations apply (21 CFR 801.150(e)).

Intentional tampering is not one of the customary conditions that manufacturers are required to anticipate.

23.11 Handling, Storage, Distribution, and Installation

23.11.1 Requirements

Each manufacturer must establish and maintain procedures to ensure that mix-ups, damage, deterioration, contamination, or other adverse effects to product do not occur during handling.

Each manufacturer must establish and maintain procedures for the control of storage areas and stock rooms. When the quality of a product deteriorates over time, it must be stored in a manner to facilitate proper stock rotation.

Each manufacturer must describe the methods for authorizing receipt from and dispatch to storage areas.

Each manufacturer must ensure that only those devices approved for release are distributed and that purchase orders are reviewed to ensure that ambiguities and errors are resolved.

Each manufacturer must maintain distribution records which include:

- the name and address of the initial consignee
- the identification and quantity of devices shipped
- the date shipped
- any control number(s) used.

Each manufacturer of a device requiring installation must establish and maintain adequate installation and inspection instructions and, where appropriate, test procedures.

The person installing the device must document the inspection and any test results to demonstrate proper installation.

23.11.2 Compliance

Where needed, instructions must be supplied with the product so it can be properly installed. Installers must be trained to perform any tests that may be required upon installation. These requirements apply regardless of whether the installer is an employee of the manufacturer or a contractor.

When an installer is affiliated with the manufacturer, records of the installation should be left by the manufacturer, but the FDA does not expect manufacturers to retain copies of records when installations are performed by third parties. In such cases, the third party is obligated to keep the necessary records.

23.12 Records

23.12.1 Requirements

All records required by this section must be maintained at the manufacturing establishment or other location that is reasonably accessible to the responsible officials of the manufacturer and to employees of the FDA.

Any records stored in automated data processing systems must be backed up.

Records deemed confidential by the manufacturer may be marked to aid the FDA in determining whether information in those records may be disclosed.

All records must be retained for a period of time equivalent to the design and expected life of the device.

The Device Master Record for each type of device must include or refer to the location of the following information:

- device specifications, including appropriate drawings, composition, formulation, component specifications, and software specifications
- production process specifications, including the appropriate equipment specifications, production methods, production procedures, and production environment specifications

- quality assurance procedures and specifications, including acceptance criteria and the quality assurance equipment used
- packaging and labeling specifications, including methods and processes used
- installation, maintenance, and servicing procedures and methods.

The Device History Record must include or refer to the location of the following information:

- the dates of manufacture
- the quantity manufactured
- the quantity released for distribution
- the acceptance records which demonstrate that the device is manufactured in accordance with the Device Master Record
- the primary identification label and labeling used for each production unit
- any device identification(s) and control number(s) used.

Each manufacturer must establish and maintain procedures for receiving, reviewing, and evaluating complaints by a formally designated unit. Such procedures must ensure that:

- all complaints are processed in a uniform and timely manner
- oral complaints are documented.

Each manufacturer must review and evaluate all complaints to determine whether investigation is necessary.

Any complaint involving possible failure of a device to meet any of its specifications must be reviewed, evaluated, and investigated, unless such an investigation has already been performed for a similar complaint.

Any complaint which represents an event that must be reported to the FDA must be promptly reviewed, evaluated, and investigated and must be maintained in a separate portion of the complaint files.

23.12.2 Compliance

The regulations clearly state that the FDA may review and copy any records required to be kept by the Quality System Regulations, with the exception of records documenting management review, internal audits, or supplier audits. Manufacturers may mark such records as confidential, but the FDA will make its own determination as to whether confidentiality may be maintained.

The precise contents of the Device Master Record, Device History Record, and Quality System Record are also laid out in this section. It is important to note that the required documents do not themselves have to be contained in such records. An index referring to their actual location will suffice. All such records must be maintained at the manufacturing establishment or other location that is reasonably accessible to responsible officials of the manufacturers and to the FDA.

Foreign manufacturers must store all complaints received about their products either at some location within the United States where they regularly keep records or at a location of their initial distributor.

23.13 Servicing

23.13.1 Requirements

Each manufacturer must establish and maintain instructions and procedures for servicing.

Each manufacturer must analyze service reports with appropriate statistical methodology.

Each manufacturer who receives a service report that represents an event which must be reported to the FDA must automatically consider the report a complaint.

Service reports must be documented.

23.13.2 Compliance

All service reports must include:

- the name of the device serviced
- any device identification
- the date the service was performed
- the individual(s) servicing the device
- the service performed
- the test and inspection data.

References

Dash, Glenn, "CGMPs for Medical Device Manufacturers," in *Compliance Engineering.* Volume 14, Number 2, March-April, 1997.

Dash, Glenn, "Current Good Manufacturing Practices for Medical Device Manufacturers," in *Compliance Engineering.* Volume 14, Number 3, May-June, 1997.

European Committee for Standardization, "Quality Systems--Medical Devices--Particular Requirements for the Application of EN 29001, " *European Norm 46001*, Brussels, European Committee for Standardization, 1996.

Food and Drug Administration, "Medical Devices; Current Good Manufacturing Practice (CGMP) Final Rule; Quality System Regulation," *Federal Register.* October 7, 1996.

Food and Drug Administration, Code of Federal Regulations, 21 CFR 820, "Good Manufacturing Practice for Medical Devices," *Federal Register.* July 21, 1997.

Food and Drug Administration, "Medical Devices; Current Good Manufacturing Practice (CGMP) Regulations; Proposed Revisions; Request for Comments," *Federal Register.* November 23, 1993.

Food and Drug Administration, "Medical Devices; Working Draft of the Current Good Manufacturing Practice (CGMP) Final Rule; Notice of Availability; Request for Comments; Public Meeting," *Federal Register.* July 24, 1995.

Food and Drug Administration, "Quality System Regulation," *Federal Register.* October 7, 1996.

Global Harmonization Task Force, "Guidance on Quality Systems for the Design and Manufacture of Medical Devices," Issue 7, August 1994.

International Organization for Standardization, "Quality Systems--Model for Quality Assurance in Design, Development, Production, Installation, and Servicing," *ISO 9001:1994*, Geneva: International Organization for Standardization (ISO), 1994.

Chapter 24

FDA Submittals

The Federal Food, Drug, and Cosmetic Act, as amended, provides the FDA with the authority to regulate, among other things, medical devices. The document gave the FDA authority to take action against medical devices that were unsafe or contained false or misleading labeling claims. To implement this law, the FDA has promulgated regulations that are published in Title 21 of the Code of Federal Regulations.

24.1 Registration

Under Section 510 of the Federal Food, Drug, and Cosmetic Act, every person engaged in the manufacture, preparation, propagation, compounding or processing of a device shall register their name, place of business and such establishment. This includes manufacturers of devices and components, repackers, relabelers, as well as initial distributors of imported devices. Those not required to register include manufacturers of raw materials, licensed practitioners, manufacturers of devices for use solely in research or teaching, warehousers, manufacturers of veterinary devices, and those who only dispense devices, such as pharmacies.

Upon registration, the FDA issues a device registration number. A change in the ownership or corporate structure of the firm, the location, or person designated as the official correspondent must be communicated to the FDA device registration and listing branch within 30 days. Registration must be done when first beginning to manufacture medical devices and must be updated yearly.

Section 510 of the Act also requires all manufacturers to list the medical devices they market. Listing must be done when first beginning to manufacture a product and must be updated every 6 months. Listing includes not only informing the FDA of products manufactured, but also providing the agency with copies of labeling and advertising.

Foreign firms that market products in the United States are permitted but not required to register, and are required to list. Foreign devices that are not listed are not permitted to enter the country.

Registration and listing provides the FDA with information about the identity of manufacturers and the products they make. This information enables the agency to schedule inspections of facilities and also to follow up on problems. When the FDA learns about a safety defect in a particular type of device, it can use the listing information to notify all manufacturers of those devices about that defect.

24.2 The 510(k)

A new device is substantially equivalent if, in comparison to a legally marketed predicate device, it has the same intended use and 1) has the same technological characteristics as the predicate device or 2) has different technological characteristics and submitted information that does not raise different questions of safety and efficacy and demonstrates that the device is as safe and effective as the legally marketed predicate device. Figure 6-1 is an overview of the substantial equivalence decision making process. Figure 6-2 is a detailed view of the substantial equivalence decision making process.

24.2.1 Determining Substantial Equivalency

A new device is substantially equivalent if, in comparison to a legally marketed predicate device, it has the same intended use and 1) has the same technological characteristics as the predicate device or 2) has different technological characteristics and submitted information that does not raise different questions of safety and efficacy and demonstrates that the device is as safe and effective as the legally marketed predicate device. Figure 24-1 is an overview of the substantial equivalence decision making process. Figure 24-2 is a detailed view of the substantial equivalence decision making process.

24.3 The PMA

Premarket Approval (PMA) is an approval application for a Class III medical device, including all information submitted with or incorporated by reference. The purpose of the regulation is to establish an efficient and thorough device review process to facilitate the approval of PMAs for devices that have been shown to be safe and effective for their intended use and that otherwise meet the statutory criteria for approval, while ensuring the disapproval of PMAs for devices that have not been shown to be safe and effective or that do not otherwise meet the statutory criteria for approval.

The first step in the PMA process is the filing of the investigational device exemption (IDE) application for significant risk devices. The IDE is reviewed by the FDA and once accepted, the sponsor can proceed with clinical trials.

Section 814.20 of 21 CFR defines what must be included in an application, including:

- name and address
- application procedures and table of contents
- summary
- complete device description
- reference to performance standards
- nonclinical and clinical investigations
- justification for single investigator
- bibliography
- sample of device
- proposed labeling
- environmental assessment
- other information

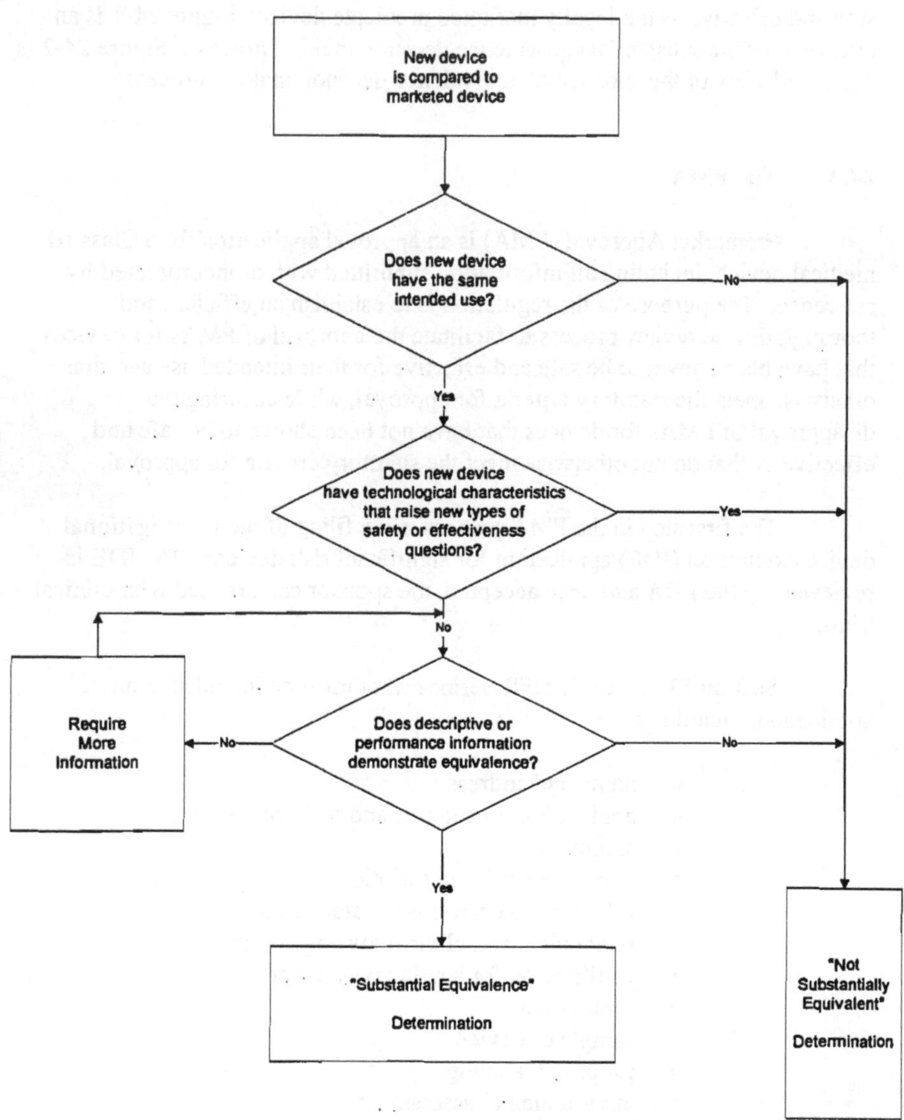

Figure 24-1 The substantial equivalence process. (From Fries, 1997)

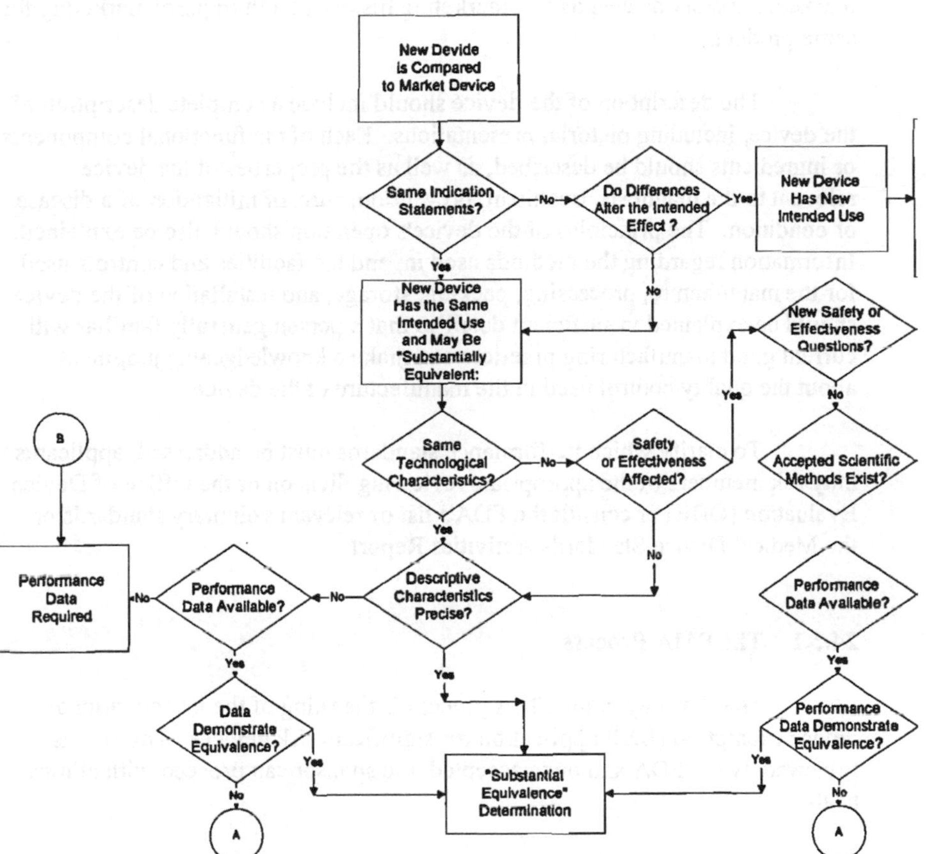

Figure 24-2 Detailed substantial equivalence process. (From Fries, 199

The summary should include indications for use, a device description, a description of alternative practices and procedures, a brief description of the marketing history, and a summary of studies. This summary should be of sufficient detail to enable the reader to gain a general understanding of the application. The PMA must also include the applicant's foreign and domestic marketing history as well as any marketing history of a third party marketing the same product.

The description of the device should include a complete description of the device, including pictorial presentations. Each of the functional components or ingredients should be described, as well as the properties of the device relevant to the diagnosis, treatment, prevention, cure, or mitigation of a disease or condition. The principles of the device's operation should also be explained. Information regarding the methods used in, and the facilities and controls used for the manufacture, processing, packing, storage, and installation of the device should be explained in sufficient detail so that a person generally familiar with current good manufacturing practices can make a knowledgeable judgment about the quality control used in the manufacture of the device.

To clarify which performance standards must be addressed, applicants may ask members of the appropriate reviewing division of the Office of Device Evaluation (ODE) or consult the FDA's list of relevant voluntary standards or the Medical Device Standards Activities Report.

24.3.1 The PMA Process

The first step in the PMA process is the filing of the investigational device exemption (IDE) application for significant risk devices. The IDE is reviewed by the FDA and once accepted, the sponsor can proceed with clinical trials.

24.4 The IDE

The purpose of the Investigational Device Exemption regulation is to encourage the discovery and development of useful devices intended for human use while protecting the public health. It provides the procedures for the conduct of clinical investigations of devices. An approved IDE permits a device to be shipped lawfully for the purpose of conducting investigations of the device without complying with a performance standard or having marketing clearance.

24.4.1 Institutional Review Boards (IRBs)

Any human research covered by federal regulation will not be funded unless it has been reviewed by an IRB. The fundamental purpose of an IRB is to ensure that research activities are conducted in an ethical and legal manner. Specifically, IRBs are expected to ensure that each of the basic elements of informed consent, as defined by regulation, are included in the document presented to the research participant for signature or verbal approval.

The deliberations of the IRB must determine that:

- the risk to subjects is equitable,
- the selection of subjects is equitable,
- informed consent will be sought from each prospective subject or their legally authorized representative,
- informed consent will be appropriately documented,
- where appropriate, the research plan makes adequate provision for monitoring the data collected to ensure the safety of the subjects,
- where appropriate, there are adequate provisions to protect the privacy of subjects and to maintain the confidentiality of data.

It is axiomatic that the IRB should ensure that the risks of participation in a research study should be minimized. The IRB must determine that this objective is to be achieved by ensuring that investigators use procedures that are consistent with sound research design and that do not necessarily expose subjects to excessive risk. In addition, the IRB must ensure that the investigators, whenever appropriate, minimize risk and discomfort to the research participants by using, where possible, procedures already performed on the subjects as part of routine diagnosis or treatment.

The Institutional Review Board is any board, committee, or other group formally designated by an institution to review, to approve the initiation of, and to conduct periodic review of biomedical research involving human subjects. The primary purpose of such review is to ensure the protection of the rights and welfare of human subjects.

An IRB must comply with all applicable requirements of the IRB regulation and the IDE regulation in reviewing and approving device investigations involving human testing. An IRB has the authority to review and approve, require modification, or disapprove an investigation. If no IRB exists or if FDA finds an IRB's review to be inadequate, a sponsor may submit an application directly to FDA.

An investigator is responsible for:

- ensuring that the investigation is conducted according to the signed agreement, the investigational plan, and applicable FDA regulations,
- protecting the rights, safety, and welfare of subjects,
- control of the devices under investigation.

An investigator is also responsible for obtaining informed consent and maintaining and making reports.

24.5 The MDR

The Medical Device Regulation (MDR), which became effective on July 31, 1996, provides the mechanism for the Food and Drug Administration and manufacturers to identify and monitor significant adverse events involving medical devices. The goals are to detect and correct problems in a timely manner. Although the requirements of the regulation can be enforced through legal sanctions authorized by the Federal Food, Drug, and Cosmetic Act, the FDA relies on the goodwill and cooperation of all affected groups to accomplish the objectives of the regulation.

The statutory authority for the Medical Device Regulation is the Federal Food, Drug, and Cosmetic Act, as amended by the Safe Medical Devices Act of 1990. The Safe Medical Devices Act requires user facilities to report:

- device-related deaths to the FDA and the device manufacture
- device-related serious injuries and serious illnesses to the manufacturer, or to FDA, if the manufacturer is not known.

The user facility is also required to submit to the FDA on a semiannual basis a summary of all reports submitted during that period. The reporting requirements for user facilities and distributors are summarized in Table 24-1.

Since 1984, domestic manufacturers have been subject to the Medical Device Regulation if they were required to register their establishments with the FDA. The new regulation eliminates this link with registration. All manufacturers of finished medical devices and components which are ready for use, including foreign manufacturers, are now subject to the requirements of the regulation, despite registration status. The reporting requirements for manufacturers are summarized in Table 24-2.

Manufacturers must report all MDR reportable events to the FDA on Form 3500A. Each manufacturer must review and evaluate all complaints to determine whether the complaint represents an event which is required to be reported to the FDA. A separate Form 3500A is required for each device involved in a reportable event. For example, if a manufacturer receives a report from a user facility which indicates that more than one of the manufacturer's devices may have been involved in a reportable event, a separate report for each device is required. A report is required when a manufacturer becomes aware of information that reasonably suggests that one of their marketed devices has or may have caused or contributed to death, serious injury, or has malfunctioned and that the device or a similar device marketed by the manufacturer would be likely to cause or contribute to a death or serious injury if the malfunction were to reoccur.

The FDA requires only one medical device report from the manufacturer if they become aware of information from multiple sources regarding the same patient and the same event. For contract manufacturers, the FDA would expect only one report from either the specifications developer or the contract manufacturer for one reportable event. Nevertheless, there must be a written agreement which identifies which party is responsible for completing the proper form.

In addition, FDA does not require that a manufacturer submit an MDR report:

- when the manufacturer determines that the information that they received is erroneous and a death or serious injury did not occur, or
- when another manufacturer made the device.

Reporter	What to Report	Report Form #	Recipient of the Report	Time Schedule for the Report
User Facility	Death	FDA 3500A	FDA and the manufacturer	Within 10 work days
User Facility	Serious injury	FDA 3500A	Manufacturer. FDA if the manufacturer is unknown.	Within 10 work days
User Facility	Semiannual reports of death and serious injuries	FDA 3419	FDA	January 1 and July 1
Distributor	Death and serious injury	FDA 3500A	FDA	Within 10 work days
Distributor	Death, serious injury, and malfunction	FDA 3500A	Manufacturer	Within 10 work days
Distributor	Annual Certification	FDA 3381	FDA	Annually

Table 24-1 Summary of Reporting Requirements for User Facilities and Distributors

A person, with nominated deputies to cover for periods of absence, should be designated to coordinate the issue of each recall and the consequent actions.

Manufacturers should retain documentation of erroneous reports in their MDR files for two (2) years from the date of the event or a period equivalent to the expected life of the device, whichever is longer.

24.6 Advisory Notices and Recalls

The nature and seriousness of a fault, the intended use of the product, and the consequential potential for patient injury or harm, will determine whether it will be necessary to issue an advisory notice, to institute a recall, and/or to report to local or national authorities. These factors will also determine the speed and extent of the action.

What to Report	Report Form #	Recipient of the Report	Time Schedule for the Report
Deaths, serious injuries, and malfunctions	FDA 3500A	Food and Drug Administration	Within 30 calendar days of becoming aware of an event
Events that require remedial action to prevent an unreasonable risk of substantial harm to the public health and other types of events designated by the FDA	FDA 3500A	Food and Drug Administration	Within 5 work days of becoming aware of an event
Baseline reports to identify and provide basic data on each device that is the subject of an MDR report	FDA 3417	Food and Drug Administration	Accompanying the 30-calendar-day and 5-work-day reports when the device or device family is reported for the first time. Interim and annual updates are required if any baseline information changes after the initial submission
Annual certification	FDA 3381	Food and Drug Administration	Coincides with the firm's annual registration date

Table 24-2 Summary of Reporting Requirements for Manufacturers

References

Basile, Edward M., "Overview of Current FDA Requirements for Medical Devices," in *The Medical Device Industry: Science, Technology, and Regulation in a Competitive Environment.* New York: Marcel Dekker, Inc., 1990.

Food and Drug Administration, *Medical Device Reporting for Manufacturers.* Rockville, MD: Department of Health and Human Services, 1997.

Food and Drug Administration, *Investigational Device Exemptions Manual.* Rockville, MD: Department of Health and Human Services, 1996.

Fries, Richard C., *Reliable Design of Medical Devices.* New York: Marcel Dekker, Inc., 1997.

Trautman, Kimberly A., *The FDA and Worldwide Quality System Requirements Guidebook for Medical Devices.* Milwaukee: ASQC Quality Press, 1997.

United States Government Printing Office, *Federal Food, Drug, and Cosmetic Act, As Amended.* Washington, DC: Government Printing Office, 1979.

Chapter 25

FDA Submittal Requirements and Compliance

The FDA has a host of enforcement options that it can invoke against a medical device or a manufacturer that violates an applicable statutory or regulatory requirement. In a worst case scenario, the FDA can ban a device. Additional severe measures include prosecutions, injunctions, and product seizures. During the course of a facility inspection, the FDA has the authority to invoke administrative detention orders against devices that are believed to be adulterated or misbranded. The agency is also empowered to require that the device manufacturer repair, replace, or refund the price of a violative device.

At the other end of the enforcement spectrum are less severe regulatory tools, such as a Notice of Adverse Findings Letter or a Regulatory Letter. These documents indicate that the FDA believes that the manufacturer is in violation of the Federal Food, Drug, and Cosmetic Act or the regulations, and request that the recipient respond with a plan to correct the violation.

25.1 Registration

A manufacturer initially registers each establishment by completing form FDA-2891. This form is available from:

Device Registration and Listing Branch (HFZ-342)
CDRH
FDA
8757 Georgia Avenue
Silver Spring, MD 20910
301-427-7190.

Following the initial registration, the establishment must be re-registered each year by completing form FDA-2891(a). The FDA sends this form to those establishments having valid device registrations for that year. The manufacturer completes part two of the form as well as any changes which have occurred in the information since the last registration. The manufacturer retains part one as proof of registration.

The required information on the registration form includes:

- name
- street address
- city
- state
- zip code
- other business trade names used by the establishment
- name and address of the owner/operator of the establishment
- name and address of the official correspondent
- estimated number of different devices manufactured.

Any changes in individual ownership, corporate or partnership structure, official correspondent, or location of the registered device handling activity must be submitted by letter to the Device Registration and Listing Branch of the Center for Devices and Radiological Health (CDRH). The letter should include the current registration number and a statement indicating that the information reflects a change in a previous submission. This information must be submitted to the FDA within 30 days of such changes.

A record of any change in the names of officers and directors of a corporation must be maintained by the establishment's official correspondent, but this information need be transmitted to the CDRH only on request.

25.2 The 510(k)

25.2.1 Types of 510(k)s

There are several types of 510(k) submissions that require different formats for addressing the requirements. These include:

Submissions for Identical Devices
Submissions for Equivalent but not Identical Devices
Submissions for Complex Devices or for Major Differences in Technological Characteristics
Submissions for Software-Controlled Devices

The 510(k) for simple changes, or for identical devices should be kept simple and straightforward. The submission should refer to one or more predicate devices, contain samples of labeling, and have a brief statement of equivalence. It may be useful to include a chart listing similarities and differences.

The group of equivalent but not identical devices includes combination devices where the characteristics or functions of more than one predicate device are relied on to support a substantially equivalent determination. This type of 510(k) should contain all of the information listed above as well as sufficient data to demonstrate why the differing characteristics or functions do not affect safety or effectiveness. Submission of some functional data may be necessary. It should not be necessary, however, to include clinical data - bench or pre-clinical testing results should be sufficient. Preparing a comparative chart showing differences and similarities with predicate devices can be particularly helpful to the success of this type of application.

Submissions for complex devices or for major differences in technological characteristics is the most difficult type of submission, since it begins to approach the point at which the FDA will need to consider whether a 510(k) is sufficient of whether a PMA must be submitted. The key is to demonstrate that the new features or the new uses do not diminish safety or effectiveness and that there are no significant new risks posed by the device. In addition to the types of information described above, this type of submission will almost always require submission of some data, possibly including clinical data.

As a general rule, it is often a good idea to meet with FDA to explain why the product is substantially equivalent, to discuss the data that will be submitted in support of a claim of substantial equivalence, and to learn the FDA's concerns and questions so that these may be addressed in the submission. The FDA's guidance documents can be of greatest use in preparing this type of submission.

The term software includes programs and or data that pertain to the operation of a computer-controlled system, whether they are contained on floppy disks, hard disks, magnetic tapes, laser disks, or embedded in the hardware of a device. The depth of review by the FDA is determined by the "level of concern" for the device and the role that the software plays in the functioning of the device. Levels of concern are listed as minor, moderate, and major and are tied very closely with risk analysis.

In reviewing such submissions, the FDA maintains that end-product testing may not be sufficient to establish that the device is substantially equivalent to the predicate devices. Therefore, a firm's software development process and/or documentation should be examined for reasonable assurance of safety and effectiveness of the software-controlled functions, including incorporated safeguards. 510(k)s that are heavily software dependent will receive greater FDA scrutiny, and the questions posed must be satisfactorily addressed.

25.2.2 The 510(k) Format

The actual 510(k) submission will vary in complexity and length according to the type of device or product change for which substantial equivalency is sought. A submission shall be in sufficient detail to provide an understanding of the basis for a determination of substantial equivalence. All submissions shall contain the following information:

The submitter's name, address, telephone number, a contact person, and the date the submission was prepared;

The name of the device, including the trade or proprietary name, if applicable, the common or usual name, and the classification name;

An identification of the predicate or legally marketed device or devices to which substantial equivalence is being claimed;

A description of the device that is the subject of the submission, including an explanation of how the device functions, the basic scientific concepts that form the basis for the device, and the significant physical and performance characteristics of the device such as device design, materials used, and physical properties;

A statement of the intended use of the device, including a general description of the diseases or conditions the device will diagnose, treat, prevent, cure, or mitigate, including a description, where appropriate, of the patient population for which the device is intended. If the indication statements are different from those of the predicate or legally marketed device identified above, the submission shall contain an explanation as to why the differences are not critical to the intended therapeutic, diagnostic, prosthetic, or surgical use of the device and why the differences do not affect the safety or effectiveness of the device when used as labeled;

A statement of how the technological characteristics (design, material, chemical composition, or energy source) of the device compare to those of the predicate or legally marketed device identified above.

510(k) summaries for those premarket notification submissions in which a determination of substantial equivalence is based on an assessment of performance data shall contain the following information in addition to that listed above:

A brief discussion of the nonclinical tests and their results submitted in the premarket notification;

A brief discussion of the clinical tests submitted, referenced, or relied on in the premarket notification submission for a determination of substantial equivalence. This discussion shall include, where applicable, a description of the subjects upon whom the device was tested, a discussion of the safety and/or effectiveness data obtained with specific reference to adverse effects and complications, and any other information from the clinical testing relevant to a determination of substantial equivalence;

> The conclusions drawn from the nonclinical and clinical tests that demonstrate that the device is safe, effective, and performs as well as or better than the legally marketed device identified above.

The summary should be in a separate section of the submission beginning on a new page and ending on a page not shared with any other section of the premarket notification submission, and should be clearly identified as a "501(k) summary."

A 510 (k) statement submitted as part of a premarket notification shall state as follows:

> I certify that (name of person required to submit the premarket notification) will make available all information included in this premarket notification on safety and effectiveness that supports a finding of substantial equivalence within 30 days of request by any person. The information I agree to make available does not include confidential patient identifiers.

This statement should be made in a separate section of the premarket notification submission and should be clearly identified as a 510(k) statement.

A class III certification submitted as part of a premarket notification shall state as follows:

> I certify that a reasonable search of all information known or otherwise available to (name of premarket notification submitter) about the types and causes of reported safety and/or effectiveness problems for the (type of device) has been conducted. I further certify that the types of problems to which the (type of device) is susceptible and their potential causes are listed in the attached class III summary, and that this class III summary is complete and accurate.

This statement should be clearly identified as a class III certification and should be made in the section of the premarket notification submission that includes the class III summary.

A 510(k) should be accompanied by a brief cover letter that clearly identifies the submission as a 510(k) premarket notification. To facilitate prompt routing of the submission to the correct reviewing division within FDA, the letter can mention the generic category of the product and its intended use.

When the FDA receives a 510(k) premarket notification, it is reviewed according to a checklist to ensure its completeness. A sample 510(k) checklist is shown in Figure 25-1.

Critical Elements		
1	Is the product a device?	Yes☐ No☐
2	Is the device exempt from 510(k) by regulation or policy?	Yes☐ No☐
3	Is device subject to review by CDRH (Center for Devices and Radiological Health)?	Yes☐ No☐
4	Are you aware that this device has been the subject of a previous NSE (Not Substantially Equivalent) decision?	Yes☐ No☐
	If yes, does this new 510(k) address the NSE issue(s) (e.g., performance data)?	
5	Are you aware of the submitter being the subject of and integrity investigation? If yes, consult the ODE (Office of Device Evaluation) Integrity Officer.	Yes☐ No☐
6	(ii). Has the ODE Integrity Officer given permission to proceed with the review? (Blue Book Memo #I91-2 and Federal Register 90N-0332, September 10, 1990	Yes☐ No☐
7	Does the submission contain the information required under Sections 510(k), 513(f) and 513(i) of the Federal, Food, Drug and Cosmetic Act (Act) and Subpart E of Part 807 in Title 21 of the Code of Federal Regulations?:	Yes☐ No☐
8	Device trade or proprietary name?	Yes☐ No☐
9	Device common or usual name or classification name?	Yes☐ No☐
10	Establishment registration number (only applies if establishment is registered)?	Yes☐ No☐
11	Class into which the device is classified under (21 CFR Parts 862 to 892) ?	Yes☐ No☐
12	Classification Panel?	Yes☐ No☐
13	Action taken to comply with Section 514 of the Act?	Yes☐ No☐
14	Proposed labels, labeling and advertisements (if available) that describe the device, its intended use, and directions for use (Blue Book Memo #G91-1)?	Yes☐ No☐
15	A 510(k) summary of safety and effectiveness or a 510(k) statement that safety and effectiveness information will be made available to any person upon request?	Yes☐ No☐
16	For class III devices only, a class III certification and a class III summary?	Yes☐ No☐
17	Photographs of the device?	Yes☐ No☐
18	Engineering drawings for the device with dimensions and tolerances?	Yes☐ No☐
19	The marketed device(s) to which equivalence is being claimed including labeling and description of the device?	Yes☐ No☐
20	Statement of similarities and/or differences with marketed device(s)?	Yes☐ No☐
21	Data to show consequences and effects of a modified device(s)?	Yes☐ No☐
22	Additional Information that <u>is</u> necessary under 21 CFR 807.87(h):	Yes☐ No☐
23	Submitter's name and address?	Yes☐ No☐
24	Contact person, telephone number and fax number?	Yes☐ No☐
25	Representative/Consultant if applicable?	Yes☐ No☐
26	Table of Contents with pagination?	Yes☐ No☐
27	Address of manufacturing facility/facilities and, if appropriate, sterilization site(s)?	Yes☐ No☐
28	Additional Information that <u>may be</u> necessary under 21 CFR 807.87(h):	Yes☐ No☐
29	Comparison table of the new device to the marketed device(s)?	Yes☐ No☐
30	Action taken to comply with voluntary standards?	Yes☐ No☐
31	Performance data	Yes☐ No☐
	marketed device?	Yes☐ No☐
	bench testing?	Yes☐ No☐
	animal testing?	Yes☐ No☐
	clinical data?	Yes☐ No☐
	new device ?	Yes☐ No☐
	bench testing?	Yes☐ No☐
	animal testing?	Yes☐ No☐
	clinical data?	Yes☐ No☐
32	Sterilization information?	Yes☐ No☐
33	Software information?	Yes☐ No☐
34	Hardware information?	Yes☐ No☐
35	If this 510(k) is for a kit, has the kit certification statement been provided?	Yes☐ No☐
36	Is this device subject to issues that have been addressed in specific guidance document(s)?	Yes☐ No☐
	If yes, continue review with checklist from any appropriate guidance documents.	
	If no, is 510(k) sufficiently complete to allow substantive review?	
37	Truthfulness certification?	Yes☐ No☐
38	Others as required?	Yes☐ No☐

Figure 25-1 Sample FDA 510(k) checklist. (From Fries, 1997)

25.3 The PMA

25.3.1 Contents of a PMA

Section 814.20 of 21 CFR defines what must be included in an application, including:

- name and address
- application procedures and table of contents
- summary
- complete device description
- reference to performance standards
- nonclinical and clinical investigations
- justification for single investigator
- bibliography
- sample of device
- proposed labeling
- environmental assessment
- other information.

The summary should include indications for use, a device description, a description of alternative practices and procedures, a brief description of the marketing history, and a summary of studies. This summary should be of sufficient detail to enable the reader to gain a general understanding of the application. The PMA must also include the applicant's foreign and domestic marketing history as well as any marketing history of a third party marketing the same product.

The description of the device should include a complete description of the device, including pictorial presentations. Each of the functional components or ingredients should be described, as well as the properties of the device relevant to the diagnosis, treatment, prevention, cure, or mitigation of a disease or condition. The principles of the device's operation should also be explained. Information regarding the methods used in, and the facilities and controls used for the manufacture, processing, packing, storage, and installation of the device should be explained in sufficient detail so that a person generally familiar with current good manufacturing practices can make a knowledgeable judgment about the quality control used in the manufacture of the device.

To clarify which performance standards must be addressed, applicants may ask members of the appropriate reviewing division of the Office of Device

Evaluation (ODE) or consult the FDA's list of relevant voluntary standards or the Medical Device Standards Activities Report.

25.4 The IDE

24.4.1 IDE Format

There is no preprinted form for an IDE application, but the following information must be included in an IDE application for a significant risk device investigation. Generally, an IDE application should contain the following:

- name and address of sponsor,
- a complete report of prior investigations,
- a description of the methods, facilities, and controls used for the manufacture, processing, packing, storage, and installation of the device,
- an example of the agreements to be signed by the investigators and a list of the names and addresses of all investigators,
- certification that all investigators have signed the agreement, that the list of investigators includes all investigators participating in the study, and that new investigators will sign the agreement before being added to the study,
- a list of the names, addresses, and chairpersons of all IRBs that have or will be asked to review the investigation and a certification of IRB action concerning the investigation,
- the name and address of any institution (other than those above) where a part of the investigation may be conducted,
- the amount, if any, charged for the device and an explanation of why sale does not constitute commercialization,
- a claim for categorical exclusion or an environmental assessment,
- copies of all labeling for the device,
- copies of all informed consent forms and all related information materials provided to subjects,
- any other relevant information that FDA requests for review of the IDE application.

25.5 The MDR

25.5.1 Written Procedures

Manufacturers must establish and maintain written procedures for implementation of the MDR regulation. These procedures should include internal systems that:

- provide for timely and effective identification, communication and evaluation of adverse events,
- provide a standardized review process and procedures for determining whether or not an event is reportable,
- provide procedures to ensure the timely transmission of complete reports.

These procedures should also include documentation and record keeping requirements for:

- information that was evaluated to determine if an event was reportable,
- all medical device reports and information submitted to the FDA,
- any information that was evaluated during preparation of annual certification report(s),
- systems that ensure access to information that facilitates timely follow up and inspection by the FDA.

25.5.2 Types of MDR Reports

There are five (5) types of MDR reports that the FDA requires the manufacturer to submit. Each type of report is to be submitted with the mandatory time frame by completing the appropriate form. MDR reports for manufacturers include:

- 30-day report
- 5-day report
- baseline report
- supplemental report
- annual certification.

Manufacturers are required to submit an individual adverse event report to the FDA within 30 calendar days after becoming aware of a reportable death, serious injury, or malfunction. The 30-day time frame begins the day after receipt of the information that reasonably suggests that an MDR reportable event has occurred. Manufacturers may receive complaint information via telephone, facsimile, written correspondence, sales representative report, service representative report, scientific article review, internal analyses, or direct FDA contact. The manufacturer should ensure that marketing, sales, engineering, manufacturing, regulatory, installation, and service personnel are trained to properly identify and report complaints.

Upon receiving information about an MDR reportable event, a manufacturer must submit a 5-day report within five (5) work days after becoming aware that a reportable event necessitates remedial action to prevent an unreasonable risk of substantial harm to public health, or becoming aware of an MDR reportable event from which FDA has made a written request for the submission of a 5-day report involving a particular type of medical device or type of event. The 5-day time frame for remedial action begins the day after any employee with management or supervisory responsibilities over persons with regulatory, scientific, or technical responsibilities becomes aware that a reportable event has occurred. The 5-day time frame for reports requested by the FDA begins when any employee of the manufacturer becomes aware that a reportable event has occurred.

Manufacturers must submit a baseline report accompanying the 30-day or 5-day report when an event involving the device model or device family is reported for the first time. The basic device information included in this report includes:

- brand name
- device family designation
- model number
- catalog number
- any other device identification number
- shelf life/expected life information.

An annual update to a baseline report must be submitted at the same time the firm's annual registration is required. The annual update does not have to be submitted if, during the previous 12 month period, there were no MDR reportable adverse events filed for the current model(s) or for any new model(s) that may have been added to the initial baseline report during that designated time period and there were no changes in the information previously submitted.

Manufacturers must submit a supplemental report if they obtain additional information denoted as unknown or not available on the original 30-day or 5-day MDR reports. Additionally, a supplemental report is required when new facts prompt the manufacturer to alter any information submitted in the original MDR report. The supplemental information must be submitted within 30 calendar days following receipt of the information.

Manufacturers must certify that they did file a certain number of MDR reports in the previous 12 months or they did not file any reports.

25.5.3 Where to Submit Reports

All MDR reports should be sent to:

Food and Drug Administration
Center for Devices and Radiological Health
Medical Device Reporting
P.O. Box 3002
Rockville, MD 20847-3002

The FDA will accept more than one type of report per envelope. If multiple types of reports are enclosed, the envelope should be labeled indicating each type of report enclosed. In addition, any MDR report may be faxed to FDA following approval. A request for approval of facsimile reports can be obtained by calling 301-594-3886.

To ensure the proper processing of all reports, the outside of the envelope must be labeled in a specific manner. The mailing and labeling requirements are listed in Table 25-1.

25.6 Recalls

The procedures for generating, authorizing, and issuing an advisory notice or recall should specify:

Type of MDR Report	Identification to be located in the Lower Left Corner of the Envelope, above the Bar Code Level
30-day report	30-day Manufacturer Report
5-day report	5-day Report
Baseline report	Baseline Report or Annual/Interim Update-Baseline Report
Supplemental report	Manufacturer Supplemental Report
Annual certification	Manufacturer Annual Certification Report

Table 25-1 Exact Wording for an MDR Report Mailing Envelope

- the management arrangements that enable the procedure to be activated, even in the absence of key personnel
- the level of management that determines that the procedure should be initiated
- the method of determining the affected products
- the possible necessity to report to local or national authorities the points of contact and methods of communication between the supplier and national authorities.

An advisory notice or recall should provide:

- the description of the medical device and model designation
- the serial numbers or other identification of the medical devices concerned
- the reason for the issue of the notice/recall
- advice of possible hazards and consequent action to be taken.

The progress of a recall should be monitored and the amounts of product received should be reconciled.

References

Basile, Edward M., "Overview of Current FDA Requirements for Medical Devices," in *The Medical Device Industry: Science, Technology, and Regulation in a Competitive Environment.* New York: Marcel Dekker, Inc., 1990.

Food and Drug Administration, *Medical Device Reporting for Manufacturers.* Rockville, MD: Department of Health and Human Services, 1997.

Food and Drug Administration, *Investigational Device Exemptions Manual.* Rockville, MD: Department of Health and Human Services, 1996.

Food and Drug Administration, *Everything You Always Wanted to Know About the Medical Device Amendments...and Weren't Afraid to Ask.* Washington, DC: United States Government Printing Office, 1984.

Food and Drug Administration, *Federal Food, Drug, and Cosmetic Act, As Amended.* Washington, DC: United States Government Printing Office, 1979.

Fries, Richard C., *Reliable Design of Medical Devices.* New York: Marcel Dekker, Inc., 1997.

Trautman, Kimberly A., *The FDA and Worldwide Quality System Requirements Guidebook for Medical Devices.* Milwaukee: ASQC Quality Press, 1997.

Section 5

Appendices

Appendix 1

Addresses of Standards Organizations

Inclusion of organizations within this appendix is not an endorsement of that organization. An organization must be evaluated to determine its effectiveness for the individual company.

American Health Information Management Association
919 N. Michigan Avenue
Suite 1400
Chicago, Illinois 60611 USA
TEL: 312-787-2672

American Hospital Association
840 N. Lake Shore Drive
Chicago, Illinois 60611 USA
TEL : 312-280-6374
FAX: 312-280-4153

American Medical Association (AMA)
515 N. State Street
Chicago Illinois 60610 USA
TEL : 312-464-5000
FAX: 312-645-4184

American Medical Informatics Association
4915 St. Elmo Avenue
Suite 302
Bethesda, Maryland 20814 USA
TEL: 301-657-1291

American National Standards Institute (ANSI)
11 West 42nd Street
13th Floor
New York, New York 10036 USA
TEL : 212- 642-4900
FAX: 212-398-0023

American Society for Testing Materials (ASTM)
1916 Race Street
Philadelphia, Pennsylvania 19103 USA
TEL: 215- 299-5400
FAX: 215-977-9679

Association for the Advancement of Medical Instrumentation (AAMI)
3330 Washington Boulevard
Suite 400
Arlington, Virginia 22201-4598 USA
TEL : 703- 525-4890
FAX: 703-276-0793

Association Francaise de Normalisation (AFNOR)
Tour Europe
F-92049 Paris La Defense Cedex France
TEL: 33+1+4291-5555

British Standards Institute (BSI)
2 Park Street
London W1A 2BS United Kingdom
TEL : 44+071+629- 9000
FAX: 4+071+629-0506

Canadian Standards Association (CSA)
178 Rexdale Boulevard
Rexdale, Ontario, Canada M9W 1R3
TEL : 416-747-4116
FAX: 416-747-4287

China State Bureau of Technical Supervision (CSBTS)
4 Zhichun Road
Haidian District
P.O. Box 8010
Beijing 100088 China
TEL: 86+10+203-2424

Comitato Electrotecnico Italiano
20126 Milano
Vialle Mon Za, 00259 Italy
TEL: 39+2+575-841

Committee of the Russian Federation for Standardization (GOST R)
Metrology and Certification
Leninsky Prospekt 9
Moskva 117049 Russia
TEL: 7+095+236-4044

United Kingdom Department of Health (DOH)
Friars House
157-168 Blackfriars Road
London SE1 8EU United Kingdom
TEL: 44+071+210-4850

Deutsches Institut für Normung (DIN)
Burggrafenstrasse 6
D-10787 Berlin, West Germany
TEL: 49+30+2601-0

ECRI
5200 Butler Parkway
Plymouth Meeting, Pennsylvania 19462 USA
TEL : 610-825-6000
FAX: 610-834-1275

European Committee for Electrotechnical Standardization (CENELAC)
2 Rue De Brederode
B-1000 Brussels, Belgium
TEL: 32+2+511-7932

European Committee for Standardization (CEN)
Rue de Stassart, 36
B-1050 Brussels, Belgium
TEL : 32+2+519-6811
FAX: 32+2+519-6819

Food and Drug Administration (FDA)
Center for Biologics Evaluation and Research
1401 Rockville Parkway
Suite 200 N
Rockville, Maryland 20852 USA
TEL : 301-496-3556
FAX: 301-402-0763

Food and Drug Administration (FDA)
Center for Devices and Radiological Health
1390 Piccard Drive
Rockville, Maryland 20850 USA
TEL : 301-443-4690
FAX: 301-594-1320

Food and Drug Administration (FDA)
Center for Drug Evaluation and Research
5600 Fishers Lane
Rockville, Maryland 20857 USA
TEL : 301-443-2894
FAX: 301-443-2763

Food and Drug Administration (FDA)
Office of Health Technology Assessment
Agency for Health Care Policy & Research
6000 Executive Boulevard
Suite 309
Rockville, Maryland 20852 USA
TEL: 301-594-4023

Institute of Electrical and Electronic Engineers (IEEE)
455 Hoes Lane
P.O. Box 1331
Piscataway, New Jersey 08855 USA
TEL : 908-562-3800
FAX: 908-562-1571

Instrument Society of America (ISA)
67 Alexander Drive
P.O. Box 12277
Research Triangle Park, North Carolina 27709 USA
TEL: 919-549-8411
FAX: 919-549-8288

International Electrotechnical Commission (IEC)
Box 131
3 Rue de Varembe
CH-1211 Geneva 20, Switzerland
TEL : 41+022+734-0150
FAX: 41+022+733-3843

International Organization for Standardization (ISO)
1 Rue de Varembe
Case postale 56
CH-1211 Geneva 20, Switzerland
TEL : 41+022+749-0111
FAX: 41+022+733-3430

International Special Committee on Radio Interference (CISPR)
3 Rue de Varembe
CH-1211 Geneva 20, Switzerland
TEL: 41+22+343-1240

Japanese Standards Association (JSA)
1-24 Akasaka 4, Minato-ku
Tokyo 107, Japan
TEL: 81+3+583-8001

Joint Commission on Accreditation of Healthcare Organizations (JCAHO)
One Renaissance Boulevard
Oakbrook Terrace, Illinois USA
TEL : 847-916-5600
FAX: 847-916-5644

National Fire Protection Association (NFPA)
1 Batterymarch Park
P.O. Box 9101
Quincy, Massachusetts 02269-9101 USA
TEL : 617-770-3300
FAX: 617-559-1849

Occupation Safety and Health Administration (OSHA)
200 Constitution Avenue NW
Room N3647
Washington, DC 20210 USA
TEL : 202-219-8151
FAX: 202-219-6064
Österreichisches Normungsinstitut (ON)
Heinestrasse 38
Postfach 130
A-1021 Wien Austria
TEL: 43+1+213-00

Russian Scientific & Research Institute for Medical Engineering
Russian Public Health Ministry (EKRAN)
3 Kasatkina Street
Moscow 129301 Russia
FAX: 7+095+187-3734

Standards Association of Australia (SAA)
P.O. Box 1055
Strathfield-N.S.W. 2135, Australia
TEL : 61+02+ 746-4700
FAX: 61+02+746-3333

Standards Council of Canada (SCC)
45 O'Connor Street
Suite 1200
Ottawa, Ontario K1P 6N7 Canada
TEL: 613-238-3222

Underwriters Laboratory (UL)
333 Pfingsten Road
Northbrook Illinois 60062 USA
TEL : 847-272-8800
FAX: 847-559-1849

Verband Deütscher Electrotechniker (DKE)
Stresemannallee 15
D-6000 Frankfurt am Main 70, West Germany
TEL: 49+ 69+ 63080

World Health Organization (WHO)
CH-1211 Geneva 27 Switzerland
TEL : 41+022+791-2111
FAX: 41+022+791-0746

Appendix 2

Addresses of Quality System Registrars/Notified Bodies

Inclusion of organizations within this appendix is not an endorsement of that organization. An organization must be evaluated to determine its effectiveness for the individual company seeking registration.

ABS Quality Evaluations, Inc.
16855 Northchase Drive
Houston, TX 77060
TEL: 713-873-9400

A.G.A. Quality
8501 E. Pleasant Valley Road
Cleveland, OH 44131
TEL: 216-524-4990

AT&T Quality Registrar
650 Liberty Avenue
Union, NJ 07083
TEL: 908-851-3058

Bellcore Quality Registration Services
6 Corporate Place
Piscataway, NJ 08854
TEL: 908-699-3739

British Standards Institute, Inc.
13100 Worldgate Drive
Suite 245
Herndon, VA 20170
TEL: 703-437-9000

Bureau de Normalisation du Quebec
8475, Avenue Christophe-Colomb
Montreal, Quebec
H2M 2N9
Canada
TEL: 514-383-3253

Bureau Veritas Quality International, Inc.
509 N. Main Street
Jamestown, NY 14701
TEL: 716-484-9002

Canadian General Standards Board
222 Queen Street, Suite 1402
Ottawa, Ontario
K1A 1G6
Canada
TEL: 613-941-8709

DLS Quality Technology Associates, Inc.
108 Hallmore Drive
Camillus, NY 13031
TEL: 315-468-5811

DNV
16340 Park Ten Place
Suite 100
Houston, TX 77084
TEL: 281-721-6600

Global Registrars, Inc.
4700 Clairton Boulevard
Pittsburgh, PA 15236
TEL: 412-884-2290

Inchcape Testing Services NA Ltd.
8810 Elmslie Street
Lasalle, Quebec
H8R 1V8
Canada
TEL: 514-366-3100

International Quality System Registrar
7025 Tomken Road, Suite 271
Mississauga, Ontario
L5S 1R6
Canada
TEL: 905-565-0116

Intertek Testing Services
One Tech Drive
Andover, MA 01810
TEL: 508-689-9353

ISOQAR
One World Trade Center
Suite 7967
New York, NY 10048
TEL: 212-432-5900

KMPG Quality Registrar, Inc.
Suite 300, Commerce Court West
P.O. Box 31
Station Commerce Court
Toronto, Ontario
M5L 1B2
Canada
TEL: 416-777-8755

Lloyd's Register Quality Assurance, Ltd.
33-41 Newark Street
Hoboken, NJ 07030
TEL: 201-963-1111

MEDCERT GmbH
Vorsetzen 32
20259 Hamburg, Germany
TEL: 49-40-369-51-7982

Medical Device Safety Service
Haupstrasse 39
30974 Wennigsen, Germany
TEL: 49-51-03-93-94-30

MET Laboratories, Inc.
914 W. Patapsco Avenue
Baltimore, MD 21230
TEL: 410-354-3300

MGQA Certification Ltd.
57 Simcoe Street South, Suite 2H
Oshawa, Ontario
L1H 4G4
Canada
TEL: 905-433-2955

NSF International
P.O. Box 130140
Ann Arbor, MI 48113
TEL: 313-769-8010

Perry Johnson Registrars, Inc.
3000 Town Center
Suite 408
Southfield, MI 48075
TEL: 810-358-3388

Quality Certification Bureau, Inc.
Suite 103, Advanced Technology Centre
9650 20th Avenue
Edmonton, Alberta
T6N 1G1
Canada
TEL: 403-496-2463

Quality Management Institute
Sussex Complex, Suite 300
90 Burnhamthorpe Road west
Mississauga, Ontario
L5B 3C3
Canada
TEL: 905-272-3920

Quality Systems Assessment Registrar
7250 West Credit Avenue
Mississauga, Ontario
L5N 5N1
Canada
TEL: 905-542-1312

Quality Systems Registrars, Inc.
13873 Park Center Road
Suite 217
Herndon, VA 22071
TEL: 703-478-0241

RWTÜV e.V.
Steubenstr. 53
45138 Essen
Germany
TEL: 4-49(0)201-825-0

SGS International Certification Services, Inc.
1415 Park Avenue
Hoboken, NJ 07030
TEL: 201-792-2400

SGS International Certification Services, Inc.
515 W. Greens Road
Suite 950
Houston, TX 77067
TEL: 281-873-5800

SGS International Certification Services Canada, Inc.
5925 Airport Road, Suite 300
Mississauga, Ontario
L4V 1W1
Canada
TEL: 905-676-9595

TRA Certification
700 E. Beardsley Avenue
P.O. Box 1081
Elkhart, IN 46515
TEL: 219-264-0745

TÜV Essen
2099 Gateway Place
Suite 200
San Jose, CA 95110
TEL: 408-441-7888

TÜV Product Service
1775 Old Highway 8
New Brighton, MN 55112-9868
TEL: 800-TUV-0123

TÜV Rheinland
2324 Ridgepoint Drive
Suite E
Austin, TX 78754
TEL: 203-426-0888

TÜV Rheinland
Am Grauen Stein
Konstantin-Wille-Straße 1
D-51105 Cologne
Germany
TEL: (+22/1) 806-82

Underwriters Laboratories, Inc.
1285 Walt Whitman Road
Melville, NY 11747
TEL: 516-271-6200

Underwriters Laboratories of Canada
7 Crouse Road
Scarborough, Ontario
M1R 3A9
Canada
TEL: 416-757-3611

Appendix 3

Addresses of Regulatory Agencies

Inclusion of organizations within this appendix is not an endorsement of that organization. An organization must be evaluated to determine its effectiveness for the individual company.

Association Francaise de Normalisation (AFNOR)
Tour Europe
F-92049 Paris La Defense Cedex France
TEL: 33+1+4291-5555

British Standards Institute (BSI)
2 Park Street
London W1A 2BS United Kingdom
TEL : 44+071 +629-9000
FAX: 44+071+629-0506

Canadian Standards Association (CSA)
178 Rexdale Boulevard
Rexdale, Ontario, Canada M9W 1R3
TEL : 416-747-4116
FAX: 416-747-4287

China State Bureau of Technical Supervision (CSBTS)
4 Zhichun Road
Haidian District
P.O. Box 8010
Beijing 100088 China
TEL: 86+10+203-2424

Comitato Electrotecnico Italiano
20126 Milano
Vialle Mon Za, 00259 Italy
TEL: 39+2+575-841

Committee of the Russian Federation for Standardization (GOST R)
Metrology and Certification
Leninsky Prospekt 9
Moskva 117049 Russia
TEL: 7+095+236-4044

United Kingdom Department of Health (DOH)
Friars House
157-168 Blackfriars Road
London SE1 8EU United Kingdom
TEL: 44+071+210-4850

Deutsches Institut für Normung (DIN)
Burggrafenstrasse 6
D-10787 Berlin, West Germany
TEL: 49+30+2601-2652

European Committee for Electrotechnical Standardization (CENELAC)
2 Rue De Brederode
B-1000 Brussels, Belgium
TEL: 32+2+511-7932

European Committee for Standardization (CEN)
Rue de Stassart, 36
B-1050 Brussels, Belgium
TEL : 32+2+519-6811
FAX: 32+2+519-6819

Food and Drug Administration (FDA)
Center for Biologics Evaluation and Research
1401 Rockville Parkway
Suite 200 N
Rockville, Maryland 20852 USA
TEL : 301-496-3556
FAX: 301-402-0763

Food and Drug Administration (FDA)
Center for Devices and Radiological Health
1390 Piccard Drive
Rockville, Maryland 20850 USA
TEL : 301-443-4690
FAX: 301-594-1320

Food and Drug Administration (FDA)
Center for Drug Evaluation and Research
5600 Fishers Lane
Rockville, Maryland 20857 USA
TEL : 301-443-2894
FAX: 301-443-2763

Food and Drug Administration (FDA)
Office of Health Technology Assessment
Agency for Health Care Policy & Research
6000 Executive Boulevard
Suite 309
Rockville, Maryland 20852 USA
TEL: 301-594-4023

Japanese Standards Association (JSA)
1-24 Akasaka 4, Minato-ku
Tokyo 107, Japan
TEL: 81+3+583-8001

Occupation Safety and Health Administration (OSHA)
200 Constitution Avenue NW
Room N3647
Washington, DC 20210 USA
TEL : 202-219-8151
FAX: 202-219-6064

Österreichisches Normungsinstitut (ON)
Heinestrasse 38
Postfach 130
A-1021 Wien, Austria
TEL: 43+1+213-00

Russian Scientific & Research Institute for Medical Engineering
Russian Public Health Ministry. EKRAN
3 Kasatkina Street
Moscow 129301 Russia
FAX: 7+095+187-3734

RWTÜV e.V.
Steubenstr. 53
45138 Essen
Germany
TEL: 4 49(0)201-825-0

TÜV Rheinland
Am Grauen Stein
Konstantin-Wille-Straße 1
D-51105 Cologne
Germany
TEL: (+22/1) 806-82

Verband Deütscher Electrotechniker (DKE)
Stresemannallee 15
D-6000 Frankfurt am Main 70, West Germany
TEL: 49+ 69+ 63080

Appendix 4

Addresses of FDA Offices

Inclusion of organizations within this appendix is not an endorsement of that organization. An organization must be evaluated to determine its effectiveness for the individual company.

Food and Drug Administration
Center for Biologics Evaluation and Research
1401 Rockville Parkway
Suite 200 N
Rockville, Maryland 20852 USA

Food and Drug Administration
Center for Devices and Radiological Health
9200 Corporate Boulevard
Rockville, MD 20850

Food and Drug Administration
Center for Devices and Radiological Health
2094 & 2098 Gaither Road
Rockville, MD 20850

Food and Drug Administration
Center for Devices and Radiological Health
1350 Piccard Drive
Rockville, MD 20850

Food and Drug Administration
Center for Devices and Radiological Health
Technical Center
16071 Industrial Drive
Rockville, MD 20850

Food and Drug Administration
Health and Human Services
228 Walnut Street
Harrisburg, PA 17108-9998

Food and Drug Administration
Office of Health Technology Assessment
Agency for Health Care Policy & Research
6000 Executive Boulevard
Suite 309
Rockville, Maryland 20852 USA

Food and Drug Administration
Office of Science and Technology
12720 Twinbrook Parkway
Rockville, MD 20857

Food and Drug Administration
Office of Science and Technology
12709 & 12721 Twinbrook Parkway
Rockville, MD 20857

Food and Drug Administration
Office of Science and Technology
5600 Fishers Lane
Rockville, MD 20857

Appendix 5

Addresses of Consulting/Training Organizations

Inclusion of organizations within this appendix is not an endorsement of that organization. An organization must be evaluated to determine its effectiveness for the individual company.

AccuReg
300 NW 82 Avenue, Suite 402
Plantation, FL 33324
TEL: 954-370-6111

Advanced Bioresearch Associates
3377 North Torry Pines Court, Suite 300
La Jolla, CA 92037
TEL: 619-535-1500

Applied Quality Systems, Inc.
2595 Hamline Avenue North
St. Paul, MN 55113
TEL: 800-633-2588

B&H Consulting Services, Inc.
11 West High Street
Somerville, NJ 08876
TEL: 908-704-1691

Bio-Reg Associates, Inc.
14900 Sweitzer Lane, Suite 200
Laurel, MD 20707-2915
TEL: 301-206-2214

Bio-Research Monitors, Inc.
201 Markham Hollow Road
Tully, NY 13159
TEL: 315-696-8139

Biotechnical Services, Inc.
4610 West Commercial Drive
N. Little Rock, AR 72116-7059
TEL: 501-758-6290

Booth & Associates
968 Shoreline Road
Barrington, IL 60010
TEL: 847-304-5685

Tom Bozzo Associates, Inc.
1617 Guston Court
Silver Spring, MD 20906
TEL: 301-871-1028

BRI Quintiles
1300 North 17th Street, Suite 300
Arlington, VA 22209-3801
TEL: 703-276-0400

British Standards Institute, Inc.
13100 Worldgate Drive
Suite 245
Herndon, VA 20170
TEL: 703-437-9000

CEEM
10521 Braddock Road
Fairfax, VA 22032-2236
TEL: 703-250-5900

Chris Flahive Associates
P.O. Box 63
Belle Mead, NJ 08502
TEL: 908-281-7000

Curtin & Associates International, Inc.
1200 East Street
Dedham, MA 02026
TEL: 617-329-1955

Drug & Device Development Co., Inc.
P.O. Box 3515
Redmond, WA 98073-3515
TEL: 206-861-8262

Drug & Device Regulatory Services, Inc.
701 Palomar Airport Road, Suite 300
Carlsbad, CA 92009
TEL: 619-931-4898

ENVIRON Corporation
4350 North Fairfax Drive, Suite 300
Arlington, VA 22203
TEL: 703-516-2300

Estrin Consulting Group, Inc.
9109 Copenhaver Drive
Potomac, MD 20854
TEL: 301-279-2899

Excel Partnership, Inc
75 Glen Road
Sandy Hook, CT 06482
TEL: 203-426-3281

EXPERTech Associates, Inc.
100 Main Street, Suite 120
Concord, MA 01742
TEL: 508-371-0066

International Regulatory Consultants, LC
2471 East Shadow Wood Circle
P.O. Box 17801
Salt Lake City, UT 84117-0801
TEL: 801-272-3550

Intertek Testing Services
One Tech Drive
Andover, MA 01810
TEL: 508-689-9353

ISORel, Inc.
5799 Auburn Drive
Madison, WI 53711
TEL: 608-273-1505

I-SYS
2772 St. Johns Avenue
Highland Park, IL 60035-1450
TEL: 847-926-0771

Kamm & Associates
P.O. Box 7007
Deerfield, IL 60015
TEL: 847-374-1727

Kemper-Masterson, Inc.
375 Concord Avenue
Belmont, MA 02178
TEL: 617-484-9920

Kross, Inc.
146 Flanders Drive
Hillsborough, NJ 08876-4656
TEL: 908-359-1367

Kuhn Med-Tech
27128-B Paseo Espada, Suite 623
San Juan Capistrano, CA 92675
TEL: 714-496-3500

Logicon RDA Quality Improvement Services
105 East Vermijo
Suite 450
Colorado Springs, CO 80903
TEL: 800-732-0037

McCarthy Consultant Services, Inc.
1151 Gorham Street, Unit #8
Newmarket, Ontario
L3Y 7V1
Canada
TEL: 905-836-0033

C.L. McIntosh & Associates, Inc.
12300 Twimbrook Parkway, Suite 625
Rockville, MD 20852
301-770-9590
Medical Device Consultants, Inc.
49 Plain Street
North Attelboro, MA 02760
TEL: 508-643-0434

Medical Device Safety Service
Haupstrasse 39
D-30974 Wennigsen
Germany
TEL: 49 5103 939 430

Medical Industries Corporation
4-2-1 Yushima
Bunkyo-ku
Tokyo 113
Japan
TEL: 81 3 3818 8575

MET Laboratories, Inc.
914 W. Patapsco Avenue
Baltimore, MD 21230
TEL: 410-354-3300

META Solutions
161 Washington Valley Road, Suite 201
Warren, NJ 07059
TEL: 908-356-9125

Microbiological Associates, Inc.
9900 Blackwell Road
Rockville, MD 20850
TEL: 301-738-1036

NJC Enterprises, Ltd
P.O. Box 14145
Research Triangle Park, NC 27709
TEL: 919-549-4100

Noblitta & Rueland
5405 Alton Parkway, Suite A530
Irvine, CA 92604
TEL: 714-258-4646

Phoenix Regulatory Associates, Ltd.
21525 Ridgetop Circle, Suite 240
Sterling, VA 20166
TEL: 703-406-0906

Promedt Consulting GmbH
Kleiner Moorweg 4
D-25436 Tornesch
Germany
TEL: 49 4122 51009

Quintiles BRI
P.O. Box 13979
Research Triangle Park, NC 27709-3979
TEL: 919-941-2888

Quintiles Medical Technology Consultants
15825 Shady Grove Road
Suite 130
Rockville, MD 20850
TEL: 301-548-0500

Quintiles Medical Technology Consultants
Mallard Court
Market Square
Staines, Middlesex TW18 4RH United Kingdom
TEL: 44-1784-461-661

Regulated Technologies, Incorporated
P.O. Box 6
Phillipsburg, NJ 08865
TEL: 908-454-2994

RJC Associates
73 Hudson Road
Bellerose Village, NY 11001
TEL: 516-437-4335

Schiff & Company
1129 Bloomfield Avenue
West Caldwell, NJ 07006
TEL: 201-227-1830

Schneider Associates, Inc.
548 Stevens Avenue
Ridgewood, NJ 07450-5438
TEL: 201-652-0706

The Science Registry
P.O. Box 784
Cranford, NJ 07016
TEL: 908-272-6811

Sequitur Associates
5 Turtle Road
Convent Station, NJ 07960
TEL: 201-644-9098

SQM, Inc.
2 Southerly Court, Suite 603
Towson, MD 21286
TEL: 410-339-5307

System Safety, Inc.
10849 Penara Streeet
San Diego, CA 92126-5936
TEL: 619-566-2556

TEKTAGEN, Incorporated
358 Technology Drive
Malvern, PA 19355
TEL: 610-640-4550

Total Business Service Center, Inc.
P.O. Box 23436
Rochester, NY 14692
TEL: 716-385-7570

The Victoria Group, Inc.
10340 Democracy Lane
Suite 204
Fairfax, VA 22030
TEL: 703-691-8484

Appendix 6

Addresses of Testing Organizations

Inclusion of organizations within this appendix is not an endorsement of that organization. An organization must be evaluated to determine its effectiveness for the individual company.

Applied Quality Systems, Inc.
2595 Hamline Avenue North
St. Paul, MN 55113
TEL: 800-633-2588

Bio-Reg Associates, Inc.
14900 Sweitzer Lane, Suite 200
Laurel, MD 20707-2915
TEL: 301-206-2214

Bio-Research Monitors, Inc.
201 Markham Hollow Road
Tully, NY 13159
TEL: 315-696-8139

Booth & Associates
968 Shoreline Road
Barrington, IL 60010
TEL: 847-304-5685

BRI Quintiles
1300 North 17th Street, Suite 300
Arlington, VA 22209-3801
TEL: 703-276-0400

Excel Partnership, Inc.
75 Glen Road
Sandy Hook, CT 06482
TEL: 203-426-3281

EXPERTech Associates, Inc.
100 Main Street, Suite 120
Concord, MA 01742
TEL: 508-371-0066

Intertek Testing Services
One Tech Drive
Andover, MA 01810
TEL: 508-689-9353

I-SYS
2772 St. Johns Avenue
Highland Park, IL 60035-1450
TEL: 847-926-0771

Kross, Inc.
146 Flanders Drive
Hillsborough, NJ 08876-4656
TEL: 908-359-1367

Kuhn Med-Tech
27128-B Paseo Espada, Suite 623
San Juan Capistrano, CA 92675
TEL: 714-496-3500

Logicon RDA Quality Improvement Services
105 East Vermijo
Suite 450
Colorado Springs, CO 80903
TEL: 800-732-0037

MET Laboratories, Inc.
914 W. Patapsco Avenue
Baltimore, MD 21230
TEL: 410-354-3300

META Solutions
161 Washington Valley Road, Suite 201
Warren, NJ 07059
TEL: 908-356-9125

Microbiological Associates, Inc.
9900 Blackwell Road
Rockville, MD 20850
TEL: 301-738-1036

Noblitta & Rueland
5405 Alton Parkway, Suite A530
Irvine, CA 92604
TEL: 714-258-4646

Quintiles BRI
P.O. Box 13979
Research Triangle Park, NC 27709-3979
TEL: 919-941-2888

SQM, Inc.
2 Southerly Court, Suite 603
Towson, MD 21286
TEL: 10-339-5307

TEKTAGEN, Incorporated
358 Technology Drive
Malvern, PA 19355
TEL: 610-640-4550

Total Business Service Center, Inc.
P.O. Box 23436
Rochester, NY 14692
TEL: 716-385-7570

Appendix 7

Glossary

Acceptable Quality Level (AQL)

The maximum percent defective that, for the purpose of sampling inspection, can be considered satisfactory for a process average.

Acceptance

Sign-off by the purchaser.

Accessible-Parts Voltage

The voltage present on any accessible part, including parts covered by service or access doors.

Applied-Part Leakage

Commonly known as patient lead leakage; the leakage that flows from or into an applied part or between applied parts.

Archiving

The process of establishing and maintaining copies of controlled items such that previous items, baselines and configurations, can be re-established should there be a loss or corruption.

Assessment

The review and auditing of an organization's Quality Management System to determine that it meets the requirements of the standards, that it is implemented, and that it is effective.

Auditee

An organization to be audited.

Auditor

A person who has the qualifications to perform quality audits.

ANSI

American National Standards Institute.

Basic Safety

Protection against direct physical hazards when medical electrical equipment is used under normal or other reasonably foreseeable conditions.

CE Mark

European Community mark. This mark is required on certain products before these products can be sold in Europe.

Certification

The process which seeks to confirm that the appropriate minimum best practice requirements are included and that the quality management system is put into effect.

Certification Body

An organization which determines if a supplier of products or processes meets certification against established specifications or standards.

Change Notice

A document approved by the design activity that describes and authorizes the implementation of an engineering change to the product and its approved configuration documentation.

Checklist

An aid for the auditor listing areas and topics to be covered by the auditors.

Client

A person or organization requesting an audit.

Compliance Audit

An audit where the auditor must investigate the Quality System, as put into practice, and the organization's results.

Continual Improvement

The process of enhancing the environmental management system to achieve improvements in overall environmental performance in line with the organization's environmental policy.

Controlled Document

Documents with a defined distribution such that all registered holders of control documents systematically receive any updates to those documents.

Corrective Action

All action taken to improve the overall Quality Management System as a result of identifying deficiencies, inefficiencies, and non-compliances. Action taken to eliminate the cause or causes of an existing nonconformity, defect, or problem in order to prevent recurrence.

Current Draw

The current consumed by the product.

Customer

The recipient of a product provided by the supplier. Also called the purchaser.

Defect

Failure to meet requirements of a product or service.

Dielectric Withstand

The ability of insulation to withstand high voltage.

Document

Information which is subject to change.

Earth Leakage Current

Essentially the current that flows down through the ground conductor in the line cord back to earth.

Effectiveness

The ability of an item to meet a service demand of given quantitative characteristics.

Efficacy

The ability to achieve the expected result in assisting diagnosis or treatment.

Enclosure Leakage Current

The current that would flow from any accessible enclosure part if a person was to touch it.

Entity

A catch-all phrase for products, services, and the activity or process itself.

Environment

The surroundings in which an organization operates, including air, water, land, natural resources, flora, fauna, humans, and their interrelation.

Environmental Aspect

The element of an organization's activities, products, or services that can interact with the environment.

Environmental Impact

Any change to the environment, whether adverse of beneficial, wholly or partially resulting from an organization's activities, products, or services.

Environmental Management System

The part of the overall management system that includes organizational structure, planning activities, responsibilities, practices, procedures, processes, and resources for developing, implementing, achieving, reviewing, and maintaining the environmental policy.

Environmental Management System Audit

A systematic and documented verification process of objectively obtaining and evaluating evidence to determine whether an organization's environmental management system conforms to the environmental management system audit criteria set by the organization, and for communication of the results of this process to management.

Environmental Objective

The overall environmental goal, arising from the environmental policy, that an organization sets itself to achieve, and which is quantified where practicable.

Environmental Performance

The measurable results of the environmental management system, related to an organization's control of its environmental aspects, based on its environmental policy, objectives, and targets.

Environmental Policy

The statement by the organization of its intentions and principles in relation to its overall environmental performance which provides a framework for action and for the setting of its environmental objectives and targets.

Environmental Target

The detailed performance requirement, quantified where practicable, applicable to the organization or parts thereof, that arises from the environmental objectives and that needs to be set and met in order to achieve these objectives.

European Accreditation of Certification (EAC)

A body created by the European Organization for Testing and Certification specifically to recognize quality system registrars.

European Organization for Testing and Certification (ETOC)

A body to recognize any Quality System Registrar operating in Europe and all forms of conformity assessments.

European Prestandard (ENV)

A prospective standard for provisional application in all technical fields where the innovation rate is high or where there is an urgent need for technical advice.

European Standard (EN)

The fundamental instrument of European regional standardization. The EN is implemented at the national level by being given the status of a national standard and by the withdrawal of any conflicting national standard.

External Audit

An audit performed by a customer or his representative at the facility of the supplier to assess the degree of compliance of the quality system with documented requirements.

External Quality Assurance

Activities designed to provide the purchaser confidence that quality requirements are being met by the supplier.

Extrinsic Audit

An audit carried out in a company by a third party organization or a regulatory authority, to assess its activities against specific requirements.

Facility

A location, site, department, or process that is eligible or seeks registration.

Failure

The state of inability of an item to perform its required function.

Failure Analysis

Subsequent to a failure, the logical, systematic examination of any item, its construction, application, and documentation to identify the failure mode and determine the failure mechanism.

Failure Mode

The consequence of the mechanism through which the failure occurs.

Failure Rate

The probability of failure per unit of time of the items still operating.

Fault

The immediate cause of a failure.

Fault Isolation

The process of determining the location of a fault to the extent necessary to effect repair.

First Party

The entity supplying the product.

Ground-Bond Continuity

The ability of the ground system connections to handle current.

Harmonization Document (HD)

A document that is implemented at the national level either by the issuance of a corresponding national standard or, as a minimum, by the public announcement of the HD number and title, and in both cases, no conflicting national standard may continue to exist after the date fixed by the Technical Board for the withdrawal of such requirements.

Harmonization Documents have a slightly less rigorous national transposition requirement than the EN.

Hazard

A situation of potential harm to people or property.

IEC

International Electrotechnical Commission.

Inspection

The examination and testing of supplies and services to determine whether they conform to specified requirements.

Interested Party

The individual or group concerned with or affected by the environmental performance of an organization.

Internal Audit

An audit carried out within an organization by its own personnel to assess compliance of the quality system to documented requirements.

Internal Quality Assurance

Activities designed to provide management of an organization confidence that quality requirements are being met.

IRPT

The suppliers ISO registration project team. A team of employees assembled that ensure that objectives related to ISO registration are attained.

ISO

International Organization for Standardization.

Lead Auditor

A person qualified to manage audits and audit programs. Also called a Lead Assessor.

Long Term Usage

Usage greater than 30 days.

Major Non-Compliance

Either the non-implementation, within the quality system of a requirement of ISO 9001, or a breakdown of a key aspect of the system.

Major Severity Level

A severity level having the potential of resulting in death or serious injury.

Management Representative

The individual within the supplier's organization who serves as the point of contact for the registrar.

Memorandum of Understanding (MOU)

An agreement between two registrars in which they may honor each other's Certificate of Registration.

Method

A prescribed way of doing things.

Minor Non-Compliance

A single and occasional instance of a failure to comply with the quality system.

Minor Severity Level

A severity level having little or no potential to result in injury.

Moderate Severity Level

A severity level having the potential of resulting in injury.

Non-Compliance

The non-fulfillment of specified requirements.

Nonconformity

Failure to fulfill a specified requirement.

Notified Body

An organization authorized by a European Community member state's government or recognized accrediting body to conduct conformity assessment activities.

Objective Evidence

Qualitative or quantitative information, records, or statements of fact pertaining to the quality of an item or service, or to the existence and the implementation of a quality system element, which is based on observation, measurement, or test, and which can be verified.

Observation

A record of an observed fact which may or may not be regarded as a non-compliance.

Organization

A company, corporation, firm, enterprise, authority, or institution, or part or combination thereof, whether incorporated or not, public or private, that has its own functions and administration.

Performance Standards

Published instructions and requirements setting forth the procedures, methods, and techniques for measuring the designed performance of equipment or systems in terms of the main number of essential technical measurements required for a specified operational capacity.

Power Consumption

The power consumed by the product.

Preventative Action

Removes causes of a potential nonconformity, defect, or problem to prevent occurrence.

Prevention of Pollution

The use of processes, practices, materials, or products that avoid, reduce, or control pollution, which may include recycling, treatment, process changes, control mechanisms, efficient use of resources, and material substitution.

Procedures

Documents that explain the responsibilities and authorities related to particular tasks, indicate the methods and tools to be used, and may include copies of, or reference to, software facilities or paper forms.

Product

Operating system or application software including associated documentation, specifications, user guides, etc.

Program

The program of events during an audit.

Purchaser

The recipient of products or services delivered by the supplier.

Quality

The totality of features or characteristics of a product or service that bear on its ability to satisfy stated or implied needs.

Quality Assurance

All those planned and systematic actions necessary to provide adequate confidence that a product or service will satisfy given requirements for quality.

Quality Audit

A systematic and independent examination to determine whether quality activities and related results comply with planned arrangements and whether these arrangements are implemented effectively and are suitable to achieve objectives.

Quality Control

The operational techniques and activities that are used to fulfill requirements for quality.

Quality Improvement Process (QIP)

The supplier's activities designed to result in continuous quality improvement.

Quality Management

That aspect of the overall management function that determines and implements quality policy.

A technique covering Quality Assurance and Quality Control aimed at ensuring defect-free products.

Quality Policy

The overall intention and direction of an organization regarding quality as formally expressed by top management. Management's declared targets and approach to the achievement of quality.

Quality System

The organizational structure, responsibilities, procedures, processes, and resources for implementing quality management.

Record

Provides objective evidence that the Quality System has been effectively implemented.

A piece of evidence that is *not* subject to change.

Registration

Official recognition, conferred by a body accredited for the purpose that a facility's quality system meets ISO 9000 standards. Also called certification.

Residual Voltage

The voltage present in any plug conductor one second after the plug is disconnected from the line.

Retained Energy

The energy stored in any accessible part.

Risk

The probable rate of occurrence of a hazard causing harm and the degree of severity of the harm.

Risk Level

A qualitative measure of risk, taking account of both the probability that a hazard will arise and the severity of the possible consequences if it does arise.

Safety

Freedom from unacceptable risk of harm.

Safety Integrity Level

A qualitative measure of the level of assurance that a component or system will function as intended or, if it malfunctions, will do so in a safe manner.

Second Party

The customer or purchaser who, in some situations, audits its suppliers for conformity against a particular quality standard.

Severity Level

A qualitative measure of the possible consequences of a hazardous event.

Short Term Usage

Usage up to 30 days.

Sub-Contractor

The organization which provides products or services to the supplier.

Supplier

The organization producing and/or supplying a product. The organization seeking to achieve compliance with standards and/or regulations.

System

A group of equipment, including any required operator functions, which are integrated to perform a related operation.

Technical Advisory Group (TAG)

Groups composed of experts who attempt to build consensus on standards issues and then advise the technical committees.

Technical Committees (TC)

Committees that develop standards on a variety of topics, based on input from the Technical Advisory Groups.

Third Party

An independent organization involved in auditing the quality system of the supplier.

Total Quality

A business philosophy involving everyone for continuously improving an organization's performance.

Transient Usage

Usage less than 60 minutes.

Validation

The process of evaluating a product to ensure compliance with specified and implied requirements.

Verification

The process of evaluating the products of a given phase to ensure correctness and consistency with respect to the products and standards provided as input to that phase.

Work Instructions

Documents that describe how to perform specific tasks and are generally only required for complex tasks which cannot be adequately described by a single sentence or paragraph with a procedure.

Index

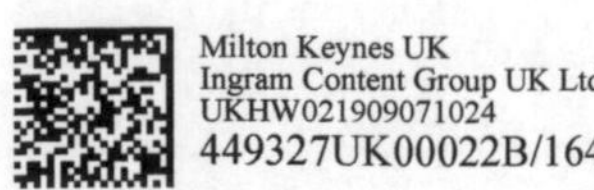
Milton Keynes UK
Ingram Content Group UK Ltd.
UKHW021909071024
449327UK00022B/1644

9 780367 400361